Uncle Tom's Hanging Tree

by

Herman P. Wiggins, Jr.

Bloomington, IN 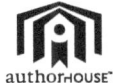 Milton Keynes, UK

authorHOUSE™

AuthorHouse™
1663 Liberty Drive, Suite 200
Bloomington, IN 47403
www.authorhouse.com
Phone: 1-800-839-8640

AuthorHouse™ UK Ltd.
500 Avebury Boulevard
Central Milton Keynes, MK9 2BE
www.authorhouse.co.uk
Phone: 08001974150

First published by AuthorHouse 6/14/2006

ISBN: 1-4259-3887-6 (sc)
ISBN: 1-4259-3886-8 (dj)

Library of Congress Control Number: 2006904647

Printed in the United States of America
Bloomington, Indiana

This book is printed on acid-free paper.

Table of Contents

Chapter 1

THE SENTENCE

Judge Green's voice crackled. Then came his piercing eye contact, elsewhere and empty.

"Herman Wiggins, **Detective** Herman Wiggins," Judge Green placed emphasis on the word *detective.* You have been tried and found guilty by a court of your peers, and it is the duty of this court to impose a sentence in accordance with the law of the land."

The Judge paused long enough to take a drink of water.

"This court sentences you to FOUR YEARS IN A STATE PENITENTIARY."

I buckled and all went silent. The judge was explaining something, but I heard nothing after ***"four years in a state penitentiary."***

I looked back at Alma, she held a handkerchief to her mouth, tears dampened her cheeks, we both mouthed *I love you.* And that was the last time I saw her.

Vietnam had desensitized my feelings. After the pressures of war, death, pain, and the pain in the eyes of children, I could felt nothing……………………..

That is, until they slammed those jailhouse cell doors … and I was back in real time mode.

There is no sound like the sound of the slamming of jailhouse cell doors. I can only liken-it-to standing two feet in front of Big Ben at high-noon.

Michael McMillan, Massachusetts State Prisoner Number 2441685, entered the correctional system with an eighth-grade education testing out with a genius IQ. Now this was a world-renowned head doctor, Dr. Michael McMillan, paroled after forty-eight years. He walked out of Souza-Baranowski Correctional Center with a PhD in Clinical Psychology, and the author of five books. One... a textbook found in many of the top universities across the country.

In one of his books, Dr. McMillan writes about "The Sounds of the Big House."

Wherein he explains the intentional affects behind the sound of slamming jailhouse cell doors. "It's a sound that says...you no longer have freedom," Dr. McMillan writes, "a sound that asks for your cooperation in making your stay as pleasant as possible. It's also a sound that says...look here you dumb-shit-head, we've got you by the balls. So, fuck up if you must, but remember, we have the power to rip-off your dick and jam it down your throat."

My cell, twenty by six feet, was located away from the general population under the east block stairs and next to the on-duty sheriff's office.

It was modestly furnished; a stainless steel toilet with matching sink. Against the south wall was a set of bunk beds, a rolled mattress, and dingy pillows.

"Herman, here's some linen," said the young deputy, unlocking the cell door. "You can make up your bed later, your attorney's here to see you, here... here, use my office."

Lewis K. Mitchell's tall - thin frame slumped and matched the long face he wore.

He looked like a defeated man, much older than when this case first started.

Lewis felt bad about losing the case, but not as bad as I felt. After all, he's going home tonight and I'm looking down the barrel of a long jailhouse stay.

"Do you understand the sentencing?" Lewis asked.

"All I heard was four years," I said.

"The judge is imposing one year per count," Lewis explained. "He's running the two perjury counts piggy-back .. and the two false report counts piggy-back.

That puts you at two years or eighteen months with good behavior."

"Where's he sending me?"

"Judge Green wants to keep you here," Lewis continued. "He's afraid your life wouldn't be worth a plug-nickel in one of the state prisons."

Chapter 2

FIRST NIGHT

After Lewis left, I felt lonelier than I had since I was a kid with no friends. The walls were battleship gray, there were no doors or windows to the outside.

The lights were bright, almost blinding. There were neither shadows nor dark corners. My cell, the hallway and other offices were as clean as a hospital and as silent as a library.

"Dinner time," said the night deputy, "come on, eat out here with us." I didn't know the deputy, but he knew me. "I'll see if I can get a table and chair for that cell," said another deputy entering the office. "We know what happened to you Herm, you got fucked and Captain Ladd asked us to take care of you."

Captain Ladd … cigar aficionado … still looking out for me.

Deputy Dave Joyden was one of the senior uniform jail officers and a member of the San Diego Sheriff's SCUBA Club; we met and dove together about two years ago on a joint department underwater ecological project.

"You lasted longer than most people thought you could," Deputy David said

"…than most betted you would," added the other deputy whom David had identified as Alvin Klinck.

"And where was your money," I asked Dave.

"Mine was in my pocket," Deputy Klinck inserted. "Some chick down in records took the pot."

"Don't call Mrs. Bacharech some chick," Dave scolded the young deputy.

"You gotta admit, that is one fine fifty-plus woman," Alvin said, looking to Dave for a response.

"She was one day off," Dave said.

"And you?" I asked, looking at Dave.

"I was way off," Dave smiled, "way off, I had you down over a year ago."

"So-little-faith-have-we," I said, enjoying the mashed potatoes and gravy and meatloaf.

"I remember your name first coming up at the department's New Year's eve party in 1970. You were the new *SUPER HERO* on the block. You were doing pretty good until you started fucking with the Doonsbury Machine."

"Doonsbury Machine?" Alvin questioned.

"Yeah, Mayor Dwayne David Doones' Machine," Dave answered, "...great day for San Diego the day Herm brought that house of cards down, but too many heads rolled from the top. I'm surprised you're still standing ... you were walking in some shitty waters."

"They almost took you out on Imperial Avenue, didn't they?" added Alvin. "Word had it somebody wanted to lamb-you-out, you must've seen it coming!"

"He's a Boy Scout," Dave said, not missing a beat.

"Boy Scout?" Alvin looked puzzled.

"Herman here believes in the American flag, a trusting government, Mom's apple pie, and Chevrolet."

"Not anymore," I said. "I still eat Mom's apple pie, but drives a British made car now ...as for the trust in my government ...

I can't give up on that … our government has its problems, but … it's the best in the world. I'll never give her up."

"I heard you did a lot of government work around the world … didn't you?" Alvin said.

"Yeah, a little," I continued. "Our government is good, we've got some good people in there and we've got some not-so-good people in there, that's when someone has to root the bad ones out."

"Considering all you've lost," Dave asked, "was it worth it?"

"You've answered that already," I said. "I quote: 'A great day for San Diego when Herman brought down that house of cards.' "

"But what about you," Dave insisted, "has it been worth it for you personally?"

"My official answer is ——YES, I played a small part in bringing down a few corrupt politicians."

I paused, looked into the faces of my small audience and then continued, "knowing what I know now, *NO!* I would think things through a little more. I was a Boy Scout," I smiled at Dave. "I thought what I was doing out there was what the powers-to-be wanted done."

I lit a cigarette, enjoying the company of my fellow officers.

"I was wrong, the powers-to-be just wanted things to roll along, don't rock the boat. And the community…well…to them, I was just another Uncle Tom."

Chapter – 3

ACCLIMATIZE

The pounding words of *"Cold, Cold* World*" by* Teddy Pendergrass was filling the morning silence. Without a clock, one hour is much like the one before and probably a carbon copy of the one to come.

I had it good … good compared to how it would have been in the Big House. Fuck…….I don't want to even think about that place…the Big House.

I saw this old 1942 movie, *The Big House,* with Humphrey Bogart, he was one of the big bad guys in the Big House, upstate New York, he had four of his big goons gang-fuck this one guy who crossed him.

Since that movie … I've had this reoccurring dream about being in some Big House … fighting off some big - bad - brothers…in pursuit of my body.

The deputies here are street cops, to the street cop I was a good guy, not very smart, but a good guy. My crusade against the **Freebies** lost me mega points, but evolution elucidated that problem.

My cell was never locked. I had the freedom to go to the shower alone.

I watched TV late into the night with the duty deputies, the telephone was off limits, I knew it…it was unspoken…I would not abuse my freedoms … such as they were.

That is until Sgt. Douglas P. Warfield rode into town on his big white horse and pissed off at the system. The new sergeant was promised a position in homicide where he'd worked for the last seven years. He felt he'd worked hard enough for the sergeant's slot there.

The job went to another... new .. younger sergeant. THE grandson of Super Sheriff L. V. Hoffman.

"What the hell is this prisoner doing out of his cell?" Barked Sgt. Warfield, his uniform impeccable ... six-one or- six-two, not an ounce of fat, I was impressed. "Wiggins is a convicted felon doing local time, I want him treated like a prisoner, gentlemen. Things have got to shape up around here."

I returned to my cell and for the first time ... I was locked in. And for the first time I felt the lyrics to *Jail House Blues*.

Fourteen days down. . . five hundred and forty-four to go!

"Good morning Douglas," I called from my cell.

"That's Sergeant Warfield to you," Douglas responded without missing a step or looking in my direction.

"You didn't see it coming?" I pressed.

"Did you?" Douglas looked in my direction for the first time.

"No, or maybe I failed to take the hints, I don't know, all I know is ...I fucked up."

"What the fuck happened to you Herman?" Douglas unlocked my cell and handed me a cup of coffee.

"You were on your way up ... all you had to do was keep your mouth shut."

"Did you see Junior coming up behind you?" I asked.

"I didn't even know Hoffman had a grandson," Douglas said getting the coffee pot and refilling our cups. "How many cases did we work together...six...eight?

I deserve that position, I know I do."

"Where did Junior come from?"

"Traffic, he's been writing piss-ass tickets and investigating fender-benders."

"You got fucked."

"Here, here," Douglas said, holding up his coffee cup for a toast, "from one fuckee to another."

On the morning of my twelfth day I received a visitor.

"Well–well, what have we here?" Said the voice of Judge Green. "Is this the VIP wing?"

"Good morning Your Honor," said Deputy Klinck, jumping to his feet.

"What do I owe the pleasure of this visit?" I said, standing and shaking the hand of the man who had sentenced me to this place.

"Can we have a moment?" The judge asked the deputies.

"Coffee, Your Honor?" I offered, filling my cup.

"Sure, why not?" Answered Judge Green, taking a clean cup from the cup rack,

"I did want to get down here earlier to see you."

"I didn't know judges visited prisoners."

"You're not just another prisoner," the Judge's voice was breaking. "I've admired your work for many years, I know you were a good cop, the streets would be a lot safer if we had more like you out there. I started to disqualify myself from hearing your case. There are still a lot of people out there saluting your cause."

I now held my cup up for a toast, "Thanks Judge."

"You're going to be OK," the Judge said, standing. "Eighteen months will be up before you know it."

"I think I'll know it … Your Honor."

We shook hands ….. and he and his aide were gone.

On the twenty-first day I had another visitor, more like a revisit. Alfonso Payton was Lead Aide to Superior Court Judge Thomas Green.

"Mr. Wiggins, you remember me," said the young lawyer.

"Yes, you were with the judge last week," I said.

"Yes Sir, I was looking at something you might be interested in," Alfonso said, pulling a host of papers from his briefcase.

"The judge remanded you to do state time in a county facility which makes you eligible for one of the honor camps, that is if you want it."

"Want it, you damn right I do," I jumped.

"Well, let me start the paperwork and get the ball rolling, I read your record, you must be feeling like a caged animal about now."

Three days after my visit from Alfonso Payton, a Miss Sheila Jordan from the probation department came to my cell.

"Mr. Wiggins," said the plump-faced woman, handing me her card, "we need to talk about this petition of yours requesting to enter our honor camp system."

Miss. Jordan searched through a mound of papers in her briefcase, "here we go," she pulled out a single sheet of paper and placed it on the table in front of her and adjusted her glasses.

"We have two camps for adults," Sheila said, reading from the paper. "Our office shows that neither would be a safe environment for you."

"Why? What makes it not a safe environment?"

"Camp Rancho del Rasa has 480 inmates … you've had contact with 394 or 82% of the population. At Camp Pala there are 622 inmates, our investigation shows that you have had contact with 547 or 88%. Who in the system haven't you arrested? Well, anyway, with these figures we can't assure your safety." "I don't need your assurance," I said. "I need to get out of here."

"Well, I need you to sign here to show that we've discussed this matter."

"When can I be moved?" I asked, signing the paper that could free me or kill me.

"Tomorrow morning, which camp would you prefer?"

"I'll take Campo del Rasa."

"Why that one?" Sheila asked, repacking her briefcase.

"I like the sound of the name."

"Are you superstitious?"

"No, but I know I'll need all the luck I can conjure up to survive."

"That you will," Sheila said, under her breath as she was getting to her feet and extending her hand. "Good luck Mr. Wiggins."

"Miss. Jordan, could I ask you to do me a favor?" I asked, holding her hand. "If there's a survival pool, could you keep me posted as to where I stand?"

"Why would you want to know that?" Sheila smiled, "as of this morning, the big money is on you going down in the second week."

People will gamble on anything.

"Time to rise and shine," said Douglas, handing me a cup of coffee. "What the fuck is this I hear about you going out to one of the camps? Bad move Herman.

I know eighteen months in here could drive you up the wall, but out there eighteen months could be a lifetime —- a short lifetime."

"I need the space." I tasted the coffee and found it to taste horrible, as usual.

"What's wrong with the coffee?" Douglas asked, reading my facial expression.

"Cream and sugar....please," I said, walking towards the coffee and tea stand, "how many times do I need to remind you ... I need condiments?"

"You're in jail, for Chrissake."

"Probably got good coffee out at the camps."

"Oooh, that's why you want to leave me," Douglas joked.

"But seriously Herman, you can't go out there, they will kill you."

"They might, but then.... surviving could be an interesting challenge."

Chapter – 4

ON THE GRAPEVINE

"What's the rush, bookworm," asked Fred Mitchell, self-proclaimed leader of the White Supremacy thugs at Rancho del Rasa.

"Loo…loo…look what Ju…jus…just came thr…through on the teletype?" Norman handed Fred the paper with his sweaty ink-smeared hands.

"You heard about tha…tha…that cop who they took down for perjury?"

"Wiggins," Fred read the teletype ……. "so we meet again…Mr. Chips."

"You know this cop?"

"Oh yeah, Detective Wiggins and I go w-a-a-a-y back."

"He ever bust you?" Norman asked.

"Who else knows about this?" Fred snatched the paper from Norman, folded it and placed it in his shirt pocket.

"I don't know, probably be all over camp by night fall."

"Find Tommy and Jack," Fred ordered, rushing to the door. "Meet me here with them in fifteen minutes."

Rancho del Rasa is a California Department of Forestry Conservation Camp.

The inmates, described as serious but manageable delinquent males, are housed at the facility …trained - and used as forest firefighters.

RDR has a staff of twenty-six - - - twelve California Department of Correction Officers, (prison guards), and fourteen CDF Conservation Officers.

All to facilitate 480 serious but manageable delinquent male inmates:

One-third: **Browns** – Mexikanemi (Mexican Mafia – EME)

One-third: **Blacks** – The Bloods and Crips

One-third: **Whites** - White Supremacy Group / Skinheads

"Just what we fucking need," cursed Mr. Lloyd P. Martin, Camp Probation Director. "We've got to baby sit this cop…. Wiggins, the one who has been shaking up things downtown."

"How do they expect us to protect his ass?" Said Jesse Campbell, Head Guard and night-stick-specialist.

"He's a dead-man, a cop off the street … in here … he's a dead-man."

"Say…man. Guess who's coming to dinner?" Fred Mitchell approached Louis Rodriguez in the weight room.

"Yo Momma and sister I hope," said Louis Rodriguez, head of the Mexikanemi Family. "Hope they stick around so we can fuck 'em."

"You ain't heard the word, MAN… we got ourselves a cop coming in-here."

"Who is he?" Louis asked, adding twenty pounds to his bench press.

"Now you wanna talk?" **Fred chitchat**

"Don't fuck with me White boy," Louis said, as two of his lieutenants slammed Fred Mitchell against the wall. "Now, I asked you a question, Skin-head … you got an answer?"

"Wiggins," Fred shouted, "who's gonna waste him?"

"Get this pale-faced mother fucker outta here," Louis ordered. "Find Cuttino and tell him we need to talk."

Cuttino Moreau, 34, spokesman for the Bloods and Crips Family, is doing time for parole violations. A lifetime member of the Bloods ... following in his father's and his brother's footsteps. Cuttino was top dog on the street.

"Whatcha got Louie?" Cuttino asked, entering the weight-room. "This better be good."

"Why, I pulled you away from that cute little bitch of yours, when you gonna share that sweet ass with me brother?"

"Fuck you Louie, what-chu want with me?"

"You know this cop named Wiggins?"

"Yeah...my man took it in the shorts," Cuttino said, lighting one of Louis' cigars, "good man, Mr. Chips."

"He's coming here to Rancho and the White boys want to off him," Louis said.

"No.... nobody's touching Mr. Chips ... he's a good man, tough cop, but fair. Brother will do anything to help you out, saved my ass many times."

"Mine too," said another Blood.

"Mine three," said another.

"No, we can't let anybody touch Mr. Chips."

"I got no beef with Wiggins either," said Ruben, one of Louis' henchmen; "he got me off on a joyriding charge two years ago."

"We gotta have a meeting with those White-Skin-Heads," Cuttino said, getting to his feet. "Get the word out.... NOBODY TOUCHES MR. CHIPS."

Demographics: The ethnic population split at Rancho del Rasa is about as close in numbers as it could be, but the one full-time and two half-time psychologists on staff log in 80% of their time treating individuals from the White Supremacy family, those fucked-up Skinheads.

"What's this meeting about Cuttino?" Fred Mitchell asked.

"This cop coming to camp is a friend of mine," Cuttino said, "ain't gonna be no cop being wasted, you get that?"

"Cause you said so?" Asked Fred Mitchell.

"No…. cause this said so," said Louis Rodriguez, brandishing the only gun in camp. "Cuttino said this cop is Ok, that's good enough for me, so hands off!"

"Not enough for me MAN," said one of Fred's lieutenants, "no cop lives in jail."

"Oh yeah White-boy, is this enough to convince you… mother-fucker," Louis said, holding the 9-MM Glock to the head of the now convinced young White-boy, "If anything happens to that cop, I'm blowing your fucking head off. Am I getting through to all of you?"

"Ok, ok, ok, we got the picture," Fred said, pulling his boy from Louis' grip, "What's so special about this cop?"

"You wouldn't understand," Cuttino said, "just trust me on this one."

"I'll try," Fred said, walking towards the door, stopping and turning to face the group, "you owe me on this one."

"I don't owe you shit, mother-fucker," Cuttino said, slamming Fred against the wall. "Touch the cop and I'll personally fuck you in the ass, you hear where I'm coming from?"

Fred Mitchell didn't answer, his silence said it all, *a cop is coming to dinner, and everyone is watching their table manners.*

Chapter – 5

WELCOMING

"Are you sure this is what you want?" asked Sgt. Douglas P. Warfield, handing me a large brown envelope. "You know what they say … be careful of what you ask for…."

"Wish for," I corrected.

"What?"

"It's wish for, you said ask for."

"Wish for – ask for, who gives a fuck," Douglas appeared rattled, "be careful of what you wish for, you just might get it, did I get that right?"

"Close enough," I smiled and opened the large brown envelope.

"It's your court orders to Rancho del Rasa," Douglas pointed out. "I have a bad feeling about this."

Douglas handed me a cup of coffee and led the way to the card table in the staff lunchroom.

"Have you thought about the possibility that this could be a setup?" Douglas asked, almost at a whisper, "I mean, this lawyer from the judge's office .. who works for the county .. comes to you with this great deal .. and he walks all the paperwork through in one day. Something like this would take four or five days.

We had this CHP guy in here for going upside his wife's head, oh…. about eight years ago, he went out to one of the camps, but by the time they got everything set up and secured his safety, the poor guy was about ready to go home."

"Yes, I've entertained the idea that someone would like to see me dead," I said, walking to the coffee table refilling our cups, "If someone's out there gunning for me, well…. bring-it-on, I'm not backing down anymore."

"Just don't forget, that bull-head of yours is what got you here in the first place."

"Sergeant," barked one of the two deputies entering the lunchroom, "we're here to pick up a prisoner for transport."

"Herman, I don't give this much hope," Douglas said, offering his hand. "Good luck, that's all I can say … good luck."

Douglas pulled me in for a big-bear-hug embrace and whispered, "Do whatever it takes to stay alive," his voice cracking with emotion.

Rancho del Rasa is approximately sixty miles east of downtown San Diego at the site of Barona Lake and on the grounds of an old 1800 abandoned gold mine. The original intent of the camp was to bring prisoners out from the city and county jails and work them in the gold mines, and the city would receive a big kickback.

"Mr. Wiggins, welcome to RDR" greeted a short, balding, plump man in a suit he purchased ten years earlier when he was thirty pounds lighter. "Step into my office."

The small broom-closet size office was neat and well organized. On the gray metal civil servant desk was the name of Lloyd P. Martin, Director. On the credenza was a family photo of his plump wife and two plump kids. Above the credenza was a mural of the **Last Supper**, huge and bright.

"A little **overwhelming** isn't it," Mr. Martin said, noticing my attraction to the mural, "religious man, Wiggins?"

"I used to be."

"Is that like being a little pregnant?" Mr. Martin laughed.

I smiled and refrained from answering, wondering how the two thoughts connected.

"We have a situation here, you have been forced down my throat and it has left a bad taste in my mouth."

I handed Mr. Martin the roll of Life Savers that one of the deputies back at county jail had given me.

"Good....very good, I'm glad to see you have a since of humor, you're going to need it out here."

Mr. Martin opened the roll of Life Savers and popped one into his mouth.

"I've followed your case, followed your career for the last two years, you were a loose cannon, I expected them to stop you, but never thought you would land on my front porch, but here you are."

Lighting a cigarette and offering me one, Mr. Martin walked over to a map on the east wall.

"This is the layout of RDR, there are no walls, no fences, we have one big L-shape dormitory which houses 480 inmates."

Mr. Martin pointed proudly as he explained the infrastructure of RDR.

"Where to put you … is my dilemma, I've been ordered not to treat you any different than the other inmates, so, with that said, you are on your own. They tell me you've arrested over 80-some-percent of these guys, at one time or another."

"Should be like old home week," I said with a nervous smile.

"They are expecting you, the word is out around camp, if you want out let me know, don't try and be a hero."

I was escorted to the dormitory by two guards, it was a cool January morning.

A brisk breeze from the snow-capped mountains surrounding the camp rendered the valley, air cold and thin.

"This is your bunk and locker," said the older of the two guards, "I suggest you keep your locker locked at all times."

"Good luck," said the younger guard.

All eyes were on me, silence broke out as soon as I entered the building, some tried not to stare ... however, others didn't bother to hide their inquisitiveness.

"Mr. Chips....been a long time Brother," said a young Black man extending his hand, "we heard you were coming ... come-on, I'll introduce you around."

Pete Holister was a small-time pimp I busted two or three times, tall, good-looking, almost the pretty-boy type, well built and lots of sugar in the tank.

He knew everybody, and everything there was to know about everybody.

"This is Brother Moreau," Pete introduced.

"Cuttino and I go way back," I said, extending my hand.

"Welcome to **my** world...Mr. Chips," Cuttino pulled me to him and we embraced like two old friends, and he kissed me on the cheek.

"This MAN is Mr. Rodriguez," Cuttino continued the tour and introductions,

"Now I remember you," Louis Rodriguez said with an unsmiling face, "you were the mid-wife when my boy was born."

"The Castellanos baby?"

"Yeah, Castellanos is my baby's momma's name."

"Born February 10, 1970, boy, 8.8-pounds, head full of hair," I quoted.

"How you remember all that?" Louis Rodriguez had a puzzled look on his face, "It's my daughter's birth date, ten years earlier. She was 8.8-pounds, and I had never seen a new born with that much hair. Is that him there?" I pointed to a picture on Louis' locker door.

"Raymond Rodriguez," Louis handed me the picture of a cute little boy with hair down to his shoulders. "Hey, Wiggins … Mr. Chips … welcome aboard, Semper Fi Brother."

"You a Marine?" I asked.

"1st Mar-Div, two years … then they canned me for getting high too much."

"That's OK," I smiled, "we are still brothers under the globe and anchor."

Louis Rodriguez and I gave the high-five and shook hands, *and it was almost like old-home week.*

"And this worthless piece of White trash is Fred Mitchell," Louis made the next introduction.

"Fuck you Rodriguez, fucking Taco-Bender," Fred snarled.

I offered my hand to Fred Mitchell but he didn't respond.

"You say you was a Marine?" Fred asked.

"Yeah," I smiled and withdrew my hand, "were you in the Corps?"

"No … my **big brother** was in the Marines," Fred said, showing a soft spot for his **big brother.**

"What unit? You know?"

"Recon, Force Recon, I think."

"Mitchell …. Mitchell? Tabius Mitchell, redneck – hillbilly from Arkansas, tall – skinny, always happy."

"You know my brother?"

"Your brother started everyone in our unit calling me Junior."

I made myself at home, sitting on the bunk next to young Fred Mitchell.

"My first time on a submarine," I slapped Fred on the knee, "your brother got me good … he said, '*Junior, when they sound the alarm and say dive-dive-dive, hold on tight, this baby goes down fast, you remember, like in that movie Run Silent, Run Deep.*' I was the only new guy aboard, and the only one holding on when the order to dive was given. Your brother gave me a memorable moment, and I have always thanked him for that. I was with Tabius when he died, so you're Little Freddy … '*Little Freddy*' were his last words."

I paused, turned and looked deep into Fred Mitchell's blue eyes and said,

"I never knew until now what he was saying, he died in my arms with your name on his lips."

For a moment, brief as it was, Fred Mitchell and I embraced just long enough to feel the effect this scene was having on the other inmates.

What a line of bull-shit … I have to be the luckiest guy in the world. I walk into a prison honor camp, a cop with a price on his head, and only by the luck of the dice, it's like old - home - week.

Well, luck and bullshit, straight from the pages of *How to Win Friends and Influence People.*

I was thirty feet away when Tabius Mitchell took one in the neck from a sniper, I knew about Little Freddy from the picture of this ugly-little redhead kid Tabius kept over his bunk. The truth is, I hated the son-of-a-bitch. He made life hell for me, as one of the only blacks in the traditionally lily-White elite U.S. Marine 1st Force Reconnaissance Company.

But … with a little sugar and spice, everything is all right.

"Gentlemen, hey guys, everyone here knows I'm an ex-cop," I thought I might as well spread a little more fertilizer while I had the floor. "I fucked up on the outside, and here I am paying for it with the rest of you sorry ass-holes who also fucked up. Some of you I don't know, but most of you I do know and have arrested, or arrested someone in your family or someone you know.

When I elected to come to camp over sitting in county, everyone thought I was crazy to jump into the lion's den. The system I so diligently served and believed in and tried to better, turned on me and brought me down. I was not smart enough to play their game. In the lion's den I'm with the people from the streets, the people who didn't stab me in the back because I have never disrespected them. I feel safer here with you than I did with those sons-of-a-bitches back at county."

I walked over to my bunk, flopped down on it, looked up at my captivated audience and said, "so here I am, back in the lion's den."

I sat up quickly, and said, "This is sort-of-like Vietnam, only this time no one is shooting at me… I hope." My eyes made contact with all present.

"LUNCH TIME," The PA system announced, and the silence was once again broken.

Chapter – 6

ORDERS FROM ABOVE

"Martin, what's going on out there?" Called the voice of Alfonso Payton. "It's been six weeks, and I expected to hear from you by now on that little matter."

"Nothing to report," Lloyd Martin answered the phone and closed his office door.

"You said he wouldn't last more than three or four days."

"He ain't who we think he is."

"He ain't who we think he is?" Payton repeated. "What kind of double talk is that?"

"He… he's in charge here."

"In charge? In charge of what?"

"The inmates," Martin tried to explain. "He organized the camp into an internal government … or something like that. He kept the racial divide intact, but now they call themselves The City. The leaders of the three groups are councilmen. If an inmate has a beef, he takes it to his councilman, the councilman take the beef to the Board. The Board consists of seven members, the three councilmen and their number one man who is a co-councilman, and get this, a Mayor…"

"Don't tell me … Wiggins appointed himself Mayor," Payton asked.

"No, he was voted in by the inmates," Martin continued, "it's like a military unit now. We have not had an inmate incident in weeks. The Board handles any problems they might have. The Mayor and the Board meet with me once a week, Wiggins is making my job easier."

"This is not the type of report I can afford to turn in," Payton said, sounding nervous and agitated, "Isn't there something you can do to. ... like .... stir things up? I need to let my people know things are turning out the way they expected them to."

There was a long pause as Lloyd P. Martin studied the words he had just heard.

He had always run a good camp, no major incidents, a clean record, and a clean camp. In fact, Lloyd P. Martin had never stepped across that thin gray line.

He'd been tempted ... the temptation is always there ... but Lloyd P. Martin has a plump wife and two plump kids to consider, so what could this nervous bureaucrat be asking him to do?

"I've got my neck on the line here Lloyd," Payton pleaded, and then shouted, "DO SOMETHING!"

Before Martin had a chance to respond, the phone went dead, and he sat there alone listening to a long dial tone... trying to make sense of what was expected of him.

"Wiggins.... get a cup of coffee and come in here," Martin said opening his office door just wide enough to get his head out.

"Have a seat," Martin directed me to one of the two folding chairs facing his desk. "I'm not going to try and understand what you've done with these inmates," Martin lit a cigarette and tossed the pack on the desk in front of me, "the conversation we are about to have... we are not having."

Martin's voice trembled slightly as he stumbled in search of the right words. They had to be the right words —- because what he was about to reveal could be a career altering decision.

"When the shirts upstairs asked me how safe you would be at Rancho del Rasa, I said you wouldn't last but a few days. With that said, I had hoped they wouldn't send you out here, but now I see that's what they wanted…. you dead."

Martin lit his second cigarette from the first without missing a drag.

"I just reported on your positive progress."

"I take it that wasn't what the shirts wanted to hear," I interjected.

"Not at all, I've been ordered to get things moving in the direction they desire. I've never had to do anything like this and I don't know whom to call or trust."

I could see the fear in Martin's face and hear it in his voice. His hands trembled as he tried to light his third cigarette from the second.

Lloyd P. Martin grew up in the affluent community of Rancho Bernardo, northeast of San Diego. The only child of City Councilpersons Alex and Charita Martin. Young Lloyd P. was privileged to nothing but the best of schools, a soft lifestyle, and class protection. Now, at the age of thirty-three, Lloyd P. Martin is facing the first stress in his life.

"What should I do?"

"Can you tell me who's putting the pressure on you?" I asked.

"No…I mean I can, but…I'm not prepared to do that right now, but I promise you I will never leave you hanging, you'll have to **trust me** on this."

Now, where have I heard those words? I don't trust anybody, dickhead, I don't know you. You expect me to lay my head in your hands and trust you? When it comes down to a head-for-a-head, you'll sell me to the dogs on any given day .. and twice on Sunday; I know you will, because I would do the same to you.

I felt a sadness .. The world I live in is void of trust, a handshake, or a man's word, or even his signature has become a mere formality.

"I can appreciate that, but what can you tell me?" He sounded sincere and for now, he was all I had.

"I can tell you that if I don't generate some action, the shirts will be doing their thing."

"Give me a day or so to think this through," I said, not sure exactly how I was going to stage my own demise. "I'll need you to keep me apprised of any directives you are given or any actions they may take."

This should be fun, like burning the candle at both ends –or - building a rattrap for a cat. Yes…. this could be an interesting eighteen months.

Chapter – 7

BODY NUMBER ONE

"San Diego County Probation staff provides programs, at the honor camps, that enable young offenders to transition back into society with the necessary skills to succeed.

The programs allow offenders to gain self-confidence, responsibility, accountability, and life-changing opportunities which otherwise would not occur in day-to-day jail activities. The programs are well developed and have had an obvious positive impact on the inmates."

— from —

(The Adult Justice Commission, Correctional Inspection Report – 1973, Section-IV, Paragraph – 1)

The programs were in place, but there were no incentives to participate.

AA .. drug and alcohol meetings were scheduled for every Wednesday night, the same time as the running of the weekly movie. The only inmates attending AA were the three or four who were under court order to do so.

Religious services were held every Sunday, an unbelievable 80%+ attended. Church participation looks good on your record when it comes time for early release. These guys prayed and read their bibles more than my Marine buddies in Vietnam.

Movie night could not be changed because of the movies' circulation schedule between camps. The Board did get the director to change the AA meetings to Monday evening ... participation increased 48%.

Drugs still ran rampant throughout camp, only now, organized user locations and lookouts had been established, reducing drug arrests in camp by 99%.

There's always that one percent of dumb-shits.

On Tuesday nights I conducted classes in communication skills, a two-hour workshop to help these guys learn how to communicate in the workplace, dating relationships and relationships with family and friends. We also included résumé writing, interview techniques and listening skills.

"Mr. Chips, my attorney wants me to list my good traits," said Eric Jefferson, second man in the Aryan Nation family, "What's a trait?"

"Your smile, your ability to get along with others, your organizational skills, anything that describes you," I said, typing out the list for Eric. "Now you give me some, what are some of the good things about Eric Jefferson?"

Eric thought for a long – uncomfortable – moment - before he began, and then proudly talked about himself for the first time. I typed, as fast as he rattled off positive elements of his identity.

Eric Jefferson grew up in the back hills of Brownlee, Nebraska, His parents, grandparents, and great-grandparents were all members of the 86th Jefferson Militia. Indoctrinated in the ways of the Aryan Nation since birth, Eric's views of anyone not Aryan crippled his progression in life.

"Let's take a walk," Lloyd P. Martin motioned for me to follow him. We exited the office building's back door which led to a large open field and beyond to a heavily wooded area.

"We've got a big problem," Lloyd said shortly after we reached the edge of the woods and two feet from a stream that bordered the camp.

"Adam Zaniarripa – 22, doing time for his first 459-burglary," Lloyd explained. "One of the CDF Officers found him this morning at about 6:30."

Adam was fully dressed, laying face down in a pool of coagulated blood. He had been stabbed in the neck between the atlas and the axis.

His pants were down below his knees, and what appeared to be semen was on his right cheek and left upper leg. Lloyd gave me free run of the crime scene before the local sheriff investigators were called.

"You have thirty minutes before I have to report this," Lloyd said, "I need your expertise."

"You need an inside man on this investigation," I said making an inch-by-inch study of the scene. "Got any friends in homicide you can trust?"

"Yes, one," Lloyd answered with little hesitation.

"Good, contact him .. we need to know everything the CSI team comes up with," I said, measuring and making a sketch of a clear boot impression next to the body.

"What do you think happened?" Lloyd asked.

"Looks like someone was packing young Adam's shit and stabbed him in the neck."

"Was it consensual sex or rape?"

"Consensual - I would say ... no signs of a struggle, and look at the semen drops. In a rape case, the droppings would've been smeared from a struggle."

The San Diego County Sheriff Investigating team arrived around noon. Thirty minutes later, investigators from the California Attorney General's Office and FBI arrived, and the scene was filled with the sounds of clicking cameras and speculations.

"Did your source from homicide show up?" I asked Lloyd the next morning.

"Yes, but I haven't heard from him yet," Lloyd answered in a whisper. "I need to keep your involvement in the investigation at a down-low, I don't know who on my staff I can trust."

"That boot impression at the scene is not one consistent with the inmates' issue. Are the guys allowed to wear any other style of boots?"

"No, everyone is required to wear issue boots," Lloyd explained.

Adam's death started the rumors moving through camp. I called a meeting of the Board to solicit their help.

"In the next few days we are going to have investigators crawling all over this camp," I said. "What we need to do is gather all the intelligence we can."

"You want us to snitch-off one of our own," Cuttino asked.

"No, but if we do have a murderer in camp, we all should be made aware of who it is. However, I don't think it's one of us."

"One of the hacks, you think?" Fred Mitchell asked.

"Keep that thought," I pointed at Fred, "that's the type of thinking it takes to investigate a homicide .... You sure you're not a cop?"

The group laughed and the tension was broken.

"Talk to your people," I continued, "cover these points:

1 ... is Adam gay;

2 ... who is Adam's closest friend;

3 ... who was the last person to see Adam and what time was that;

4 … was Adam chummy with any staff member or members;

5 … who did Adam have a beef with?

Keep everything on the hush-hush .. we don't want the guards knowing we suspect one of them. One other thing" I added, "is there any inmate on a guard's pay-roll?"

"None that I know of," said Louis, and the others shook their heads in agreement.

Investigating a homicide under these conditions will be extremely difficult for the authorities. Gathering evidence and interviewing inmate witnesses is just the start of their nightmare.

But I had the pleasure of putting together my own team of enthusiastic investigators. They were men who hate the system … men who hated me just six weeks ago.

Chapter – 8

THE ROLL-UP

When not responding to emergencies, inmates are busy with conservation and community service work projects for local, state, and federal government agencies. The citizens of California receive a huge benefit by housing these serious, but controllable inmates. Fire crews average in excess of two million hours of emergency response time each year, and eight million hours of work projects.

The three fire-fighting teams are pretty equally balanced racially across the line. While combating forest fires, team members have to rely on … and trust each other.

"Brother Fremin, I owe you," said Jesse Balentine, number three man in the Aryan Nation, "quick action out there, Brother, I'll save your Black ass next time."

"No sweat, White-Boy, you can be my slave for a week."

The two men from opposite sides of the track hi-fived, bumped chest, and embraced as brothers in combat do.

FFT-3 —- was dispatched to a brush fire 30 miles east of camp. A sudden wind change caught Jessie and two other fire fighters in a box canyon blocked by a 200-yard wide wall of flames. Fremin, lead hose man, observed the entrapment from a higher ground, laid down a volley of water in the center of the wall creating a path, freeing the three trapped firemen.

"Mr. Chips, got a minute," asked Greg Abboud, a tall, young brother who belongs to neither the Bloods nor the Crips, but is forced by the color of his skin to seek alliance with Cuttino Moreau and his group of merry men.

"Sure Greg, how're you doing today?" I extended my hand. "Have a seat, what's on your mind?"

"That guy Adam … the one who got killed," Greg started, nervously lighting a cigarette, "we were on the same ship together."

"You a Navy man too?"

"I thought you were a Marine," Greg looked confused.

"Marines are Sailors."

"I didn't know that."

"I've probably had more ship time than you … Kid," I said, sounding like an old-salt. "What can you tell me about Adam?"

"I think he was gay," Greg whispered. "Word got around the ship about Adam and some other guys."

"Words like what?"

"They were punks, you know…. they did each other."

"And how reliable is this word?"

"Reliable, I saw Adam and this big white boy coming out of the mop locker," Greg continued whispering, "they weren't cleaning mops either."

"You see him with anybody around here?"

"He smoked pot with Mr. Clavesilla."

"Mr. Clavesilla, the fat guard," I was now whispering.

"One of the fat guards," added Greg smiling.

Greg had a point, eight of the twelve guards had waistlines in excess of 50 inches, and the other four were pushing the hell out of the 40-inch mark.

They ranged in the age group of senior citizens. The inmates knew they could out - run any one of them ... and in most cases, a brisk walk would undoubtedly do the job.

"What can you tell me about this Mr. Clavesilla," I asked, watching the young man move nervously in his chair.

"Mr. Clavesilla is cool," Greg said, his eyes scanning the room for listening ears, "he don't bring any dope to the table, just smokes up the inmate's stash. I don't know anything about him being gay ... all I know is, he and Adam always smoked pot in back of the tool shed."

"Have you said anything to Cuttino about this?"

"No, I don't trust Cuttino."

"Why's that," I asked, canceling my unspoken thoughts of Cuttino.

"Cuttino don't like me so much," Greg said, his voice quivered on the edge of hysteria. "I'm from North Carolina, I don't know nothing about no gangs ... and I don't want to be in no gang... he keeps pressuring me to be a Crip."

"Ok, do this for me," I instructed the young sailor, "tell Cuttino everything you've told me here ... don't let him know you talked to me ... I need to see how much info feeds down the line."

Greg shook his head, but I could read the fear in his green eyes ... and in his half-forced smile.

I need to take a look at the boots Guard Clavesilla wore. The boot impression at the crime scene was deep enough to be consistent with a heavy man, but then, that could be any of the guards.

It was noon and Lloyd P. Martin hadn't arrived at the camp office. He was normally the first in every morning, and the last to leave every night.

"Wiggins, what do-you-do around here all day?" Jesse Campbell, CDF Officer, asked.. in a put-on voice of authority.

"I play the cute little security until Mrs. Macias gets back from vacation," I answered jokingly.

"I got an opening in the tool shed if you want it."

"Sounds good to me, but I think Mr. Martin wants me here until Mrs. Macias returns."

"Ok… Ok, I'll talk to Lloyd when Donna gets back .. I could sure use you."

The conservation camp program in California has a history that spans 55 years, as far back as 1915. And from the looks of some of these buildings, this camp has been on the front line since inception.

During World War II, much of the firefighting workforce utilized to fight brush and forest fires were committed to wartime efforts. The CDF and the California Correction Department joined forces to establish 41 temporary camps to augment fire-fighting resources.

"Mr. Clavesilla, how are you doing today?" I spoke to the slow walking guard, following him, hoping to get a look at the treads on his boots.

"I'm good.. young man," he said, having to turn his whole body to look in my direction. "How much time you doing, Wiggins?"

"Two years Sir," I said, almost missing his question as I tried to study his boot prints in the sand, noting they didn't match the one found at the crime scene.

"Wiggins, have you seen Cuttino?" Asked one of the CDF Officers quickly walking towards the dormitory and sounding upset. "He's been missing all day."

"Missing, Sir?"

"Yeah…. the son-of-a-bitch didn't report for training, and no one seems to have seen him."

AWOL is not much of a problem in an honor camp. Most of these guys are only doing short time sentences. Cuttino is down to 55 days and a wake-up; I can't imagine him going over the hill at this stage of his sentence.

"Louis, where's Cuttino?" I asked, entering the mess hall.

"He got rolled-up," Louis brusquely answered.

"What happened?"

"He got this phone call from home this morning, and went section-eight."

"Where is he now?"

"In lock-up … waiting for the Sheriff transport."

Lock-up is a one-man cell in the back of the HQ Office. Inmates, fucking up enough to warrant a return trip to county jail, are kept there until Sheriff Officers come in from the city.

"Cuttino, what happened?" I asked from the free side of the bars.

"My old lady's ex-husband went upside her head and broke her neck last night," Cuttino cried, "I gotta get out of here, I'm gonna kill the mother-fucker."

"What did you do to end-up in here?" I asked, noticing how cold the room was and asking, "Don't they have heat back here?"

"This is the cool-down cell," Cuttino's voice cracked with tears, "I clobbered one of the guards."

"Cuttino – Cuttino – you – done – fucked – up – good," I paused and thought for a moment, "Hang tight, who was the guard?"

"Mr. Mackenzie."

"Oh-shit.... of all people.... Mr. Mackenzie, I'll be back."

Mackenzie is the only guard that doesn't walk around with a hard-on for the inmates. Of all the guards, he has more compassion and understanding for these guys. Black, in his 50s, and a former Marine — Mackenzie works out on the yard with the inmates and seems to be in tune to their pain.

"Mr. Mackenzie, got a moment?" I asked, entering the camp director's office.

"I'm on my way to see Lloyd, what's up?" Mackenzie continued walking,

"Ok, I'll go with you," I said, and we both entered Lloyd P. Martin's office shoulder to shoulder.

"I read your report on the Moreau incident," Lloyd said, before either Mackenzie or I had a chance to speak. "Looks cut and dry to me. Wiggins what are you doing here?"

"Cuttino fucked-up," I started, "but he's a good man. Mr. Martin, he just got some bad news and he wasn't thinking clearly."

"Fucked-up is putting it mildly," Lloyd added, "these inmates know it's roll-up time if they lay a hand on a correctional officer."

"He knows he fucked up ... and is ready to apologize to Mr. Mackenzie," I pleaded Cuttino's case. "Isn't there anything we can do for him? Cuttino has the Blacks under control, we need him."

"Mr. Chips.......I mean, Mr. Wiggins...."

"You can call me Mr. Chips," I interrupted Mackenzie.

"... has a point," Mackenzie continued, "the camp hasn't been this quiet in years."

"You're willing to drop these charges?" Lloyd asked.

"Well….. yes, I think so," Mackenzie hesitated.

"How about doing it for me, Mr. Mackenzie, for a fellow Marine?"

"Hold it – hold it," Lloyd held up both hands, "if the rest of the inmates hear about Moreau getting away with striking one of my officers, it could set a dangerous precedent."

"What if I give you my word that nothing like this will happen again?" I asked, looking at Lloyd, then back to Mackenzie, "let me diffuse this Sir."

Lloyd P. Martin thought in silence … slowly running his plump fingers through his now gray hair … and then lighting another cigarette.

The walls of the small office seemed to be moving in, crunching the stagnant silence into an unbearable concentration.

"Ok…how do you plan to handle this?" Lloyd finally spoke.

"We have a camp meeting tonight, I'll just tell them how it went down and how Mr. Mackenzie decided to give Cuttino another chance."

"All right," Lloyd said, tossing Mackenzie a ring of keys, "let him out, **unroll him**, so to speak … I'll talk to him tomorrow."

Tossing me the keys, Mackenzie said, "you take him back to the dorm, I'll see him tomorrow here in Mr. Martin's office."

"Thank you guys," I said, getting to my feet, "I think we made the right decision."

"You ever think about being a lawyer?" Mackenzie asked – smiling, "you have a knack for this stuff."

I was putting together my speech as I headed to the cooling-off room, choosing the right words for Cuttino was one thing, but having the right words for the camp's meeting was even more crucial. Striking a guard is definitely a roll-up offense. Explaining Cuttino's defense, which there is none, will be like pulling a rabbit from a hat.

"Lets go Bad-Boy," I said, unlocking the cell door, "you're **unrolled**."

"What happened?" Cuttino asked, not hesitating his lock-up exit, "how you pull this off?"

"You have a meeting in the Director's office at 9-AM tomorrow ... at which time you are going to tuck your tail between your legs and meekly apologize to Mr. Mackenzie and the Director."

I placed a hand on Cuttino's chest, stopping him at the cell door and said, "you got a problem with that?"

"No problem at all Mr. Chips," he grinned, "I owe you big time."

"That you do, Mr. Moreau .....that you do."

At the camp meeting, just before the weekly movie, I made my point. Although many questioned how I was able to pull off such a task, my stock went up 1000 fold.

Chapter – 9

BODY NUMBER TWO

"Good morning Mr. Martin," I said, not missing a stroke on the typewriter, "this is going to be the best day in your life."

"Wrong ..." Lloyd said with a displeased look and sound in his voice.

"What's wrong, the wife turn you down this morning," I said, following Lloyd into his office.

"We've got another body," he said changing into a pair of high-top boots, "found only a few feet from the first one."

I followed Lloyd to the edge of the woods where the fully clothed body of a male Black lay face down in the stream. Like the first body, his pants were down below his knees.

"Look," I said, pointing to the leaves around the body, "his pants were pulled down after he was down."

"How can you tell that?" Lloyd asked, squatting next to the body.

"See how the leaves are raked back," I pointed, "like they were pulled aside by a loose belt."

"Was he sexually assaulted?"

"I don't think so, no semen present," like on the first body, I used two pencils to spread his cheeks and expose his rectum, "see .. no semen there either."

Howard Newton, age 26, doing a year for possession of marijuana, oh yes...I knew Howard, his mother, father, and all five brothers, arrested the whole family at one time or another.

The Newton family has lived in, and terrorized, the community of Linda Vista for years. Tom Newton, the father, is doing time, big time, in the big house for killing his brother .. father .. number one son .. fourth and sixth son, at the end of a lovely family game of dominoes.

Number two son was killed by the owner of a 7-11 store.

Number three son and dear old Mom went away for welfare fraud.

Oh yeah... number three son was killed in Q.

And there lies number five son, face down in a stream - what a lineage.

A portrait of the world's most dysfunctional family.

I had a strange feeling about this crime scene. It's so much like the first one yet, not like it at all. Almost as if.....as if someone wanted the two to appear related.

Related – related, that's it, look for the overuse in reverse, what are the differences?

I took twelve snapshots of the crime scene. I knew once the real detectives arrived I wouldn't have access to the area.... There it was, ten feet east of the stream, fresh boot tracks, the same markings found next to the first body.

I followed the boot tracks east then south through the woods. They led to an access road that runs east and west - connecting to Rancho del Rasa Road, the main way **in** and **out** of camp. Tire treadmarks on the access road looked to be from a quarter-ton truck heading in the direction of camp.

Within two hours Rancho del Rasa was the most popular place on earth, County Sheriff vehicles parked all over the area. Then came the DA and 16 more vehicles, FBI – nine vehicles, SDPD – four vehicles, and two vehicles marked

Treasury Department. Oh yes, can't forget the news wagons, all the major stations and some I'd never heard of.

Lights – Camera – Action. Everyone was having his fifteen minutes of fame. Camera crews invaded the dormitory - interviewing inmates about the *string of murders* in camp.

Having had my share of the lights, cameras and the media, I watched the circus from the hill behind the tool shed.

The media had its run of the camp until someone from the director's office took a look out the window and saw the melee.

CSI hung enough lights around the crime scene to render a day-like environment.

"Lloyd, here's my report and findings," I said, handing the director a brown envelope, "I didn't sign it, it's yours."

"Have you heard of a Tomika Sciortino?" Lloyd read from a phone bill. "He's been calling here...yes, twice, collect, from The California Men's Colony."

"I know him…. uhuh….I arrested him, Director of the Black Panthers, San Diego Chapter," I said, and thought of my last meeting with Dr. Sciortino, and his cold eyes. His voice sounded forgiving, but those piercing cold eyes said revenge.

Dr. Sciortino was my biggest fear. Not many of my other numerous enemies would have me anxious, but this man would reach from his grave, I just know it. I'll….I'll never forget that smile … and that look of death. He's coming after me … I don't know how, but I just know he is.

"Who's receiving the calls?" I asked.

"I don't know," Lloyd closely examined the phone bill, "they came in on an office line, between 2341 and 0015 hours."

"Whos here that Dr. Sciortino could be calling, and why?"

2200 hours – Count down – **"all present and accounted for"** announced the PA system. All the CSI's lights were off, media gone, parking lot empty. The energy in the dorm effervesced until lights out. Groups played cameramen, while others repeated their time under the lights and enjoyed seeing themselves on the 9:30 news.

"It's a beautiful day," I shouted, 30 - seconds before the wake-up-blasts,

"I'm alive, I'm alert, optimistic and enthusiastic about life!"

"Fuck-You," a voice from the north wing rang out, and echoes were repeated many more times.

The first time I gave my rendition of revelry nearly caused a riot, The wake-up blast sounds at 0630. First count is at formation on the track – 0700, then we march off to the mess hall or fall out of formation to sleep another thirty minutes, 0800 – work formation and 2nd count.

"This loud-shit of yours has got to cease and discontinue at once," said Alan Wilson, hype and small time 211-man.

"I like this," said Greg Abboud, standing in the corner of the room, "this is cool. Before Mr. Chips came here, if somebody would wake up everybody like that, he would be having his court-in-the-street .. leading to an ass stomping. But look at us." young Greg held up his hands, moving to the center of the room and turning 360° "we're talking, we are not animals, we are talking."

Greg Abboud, nervous little sailor boy being assertive, you go Greg!

He had their attention, little movement, no sound.

"I agree with Greg," Louis Rodriguez stood and turned to face me, "but come on Mr. Chips, I also agree with Alan."

44

"Ok… what if I only say *good morning Camp Rancho del Rasa,*" I added.

"Lets say, you only say *good morning,*" Louis bartered.

"I can live with that," I smiled and extended my hand to Louis, then to Fred, and finally Cuttino Moreau, holding my grip longer than needed and looking deep into his eyes, making my presence known.

His eyes were timid, uncertain, even reticent like.

"Is this all about making a point," a faceless voice called from a corner of the room.

"No, I was just really feeling good this morning," I said, scanning the crowd of on-lookers, calculating my next words, "but, we did see how nice it is living in an organized society."

It was all to make a point, calculated to teach. One thing I did learn from the Southern Baptist Church, **keeping control of your flock and provide it with the opportunity to discover how good life is with you in charge.**

Right now, my life is all about surviving. I'm prepared to do anything, say anything, and be anybody it takes to stay alive, and if I must…..**kill….**

"What are you doing in here so early?" asked Don Carvesilla, stating he wasn't expecting anyone in the office at this early hour.

"Have a lot of paperwork to catch up on," I said, and went straight to work at my desk.

Don Carvesilla left the building without saying a word. I low-crawled through the office to the phone receiving calls from Dr. Tomiko Sciortino. In the wall plate, I installed a crude recorder that starts and stops with a dial tone.

"Greg," I called to the young man walking through the workout field.

"Yes Sir, you calling me Mr. Chips?" Greg stopped and ran in my direction. "Good morning Sir."

"Good morning to you Kid," I lightly touched his arm directing him to walk with me. "Good thinking last night," I said, "what you said in the meeting, good stuff."

"It seemed like the thing to say at the time," Greg said, smiling proudly.

"It was.... it was the right thing at the right time, thanks for your kind words."

"We work good together Mr. Chips," Greg's face glowed, "can I work with you on these cases?"

"Ok...Kid, I could use a second set of senses."

"Senses?"

"Yeah, like sight, hearing, smell ... somebody to watch my back."

"I'm your man Mr. Chips, back home they used to say I had more sense than our hog .. you know .. hogs are smart."

"Thank you Greg — I didn't know that," I said, not letting him see the expression on my face.

For six days I got to the office early, removed my crude recorder and listened to the calls coming in on that phone. Nothing from Dr. Sciortino, but on the morning of the seventh day, I heard his voice for the first time in many months .. deep .. slow, well manicured words. It was him ... and I had my ace in a hole.

Chapter – 10

ACE IN THE HOLE

It was a perfect cloudless day; Santa Ana winds had pushed back the valley smog, leaving a crisp and clear dawn.

Sunday is a non-work day .. that is until the alarm sounds for a brush or forest fire. Most inmates sleep ... very few attend breakfast (which starts at 0700 and lasts only fifteen minutes). Church service attendance went from two inmates to 170 inmates. Only after the council was able to get it moved from 0730 to 1730 (5:30-pm). But Sunday morning is for kicking-back with the Sunday paper . . . a cup of coffee ... and a joint ... and your jail-house bitch at your side.

Vehicles start filling the parking lot as early as 0800 ... visiting hours don't start until 1000 hrs.

It was May, my fifth month in camp, I didn't have visitors. I guess you have to have friends to have visitors, it didn't matter, I had been alone all of my life and it wasn't bad. Like in the jungles, you don't need anybody. Like in the streets, you don't need anybody, they slow you down, and you can get real fucked up having friends, who needs 'em?

I sat on the hill behind the tool shed listening to the voices on the crude: jerry-rigged recording device I'd put together. Dr. Sciortino's voice, I recognized it, but who is he calling? Who is Sciortino working with?

Dr. Sciortino: *"Well, where are we?"*

Un-ID'd voice: *"I dropped it this time, I'm sure the cops found it."*

Dr. Sciortino: *"They'd better find it, this is your last chance to fuck-up."*

Un-ID'd voice: *"You think that coin will be enough?"*

Dr. Sciortino: *"WE NEED TO ONLY PLANT THE SEED, HAVE FAITH IN OUR MEN IN BLUE OR BROWN TO DO THEIR JOB WELL."*

Un-ID'd voice: *"What you want me doing next?"*

Dr. Sciortino: *"Keep your eyes and ears open, stand by for my next call."*

Un-ID'd voice: *"Ok.... I'll keep an eye on him."*

The conversation ended without a salutation. Who could he be talking to, and what is this all about?

I played the tape again, and again, and again, making notes and picking up a little something each time.

"Hey-there Mr. Chips," Greg Abboud said, trying to disguise a slight stutter.

"I thought I'd find you up here ... you like this spot don't you?"

"Good morning Greg," I greeted flatly, not wanting to share my hill or this moment, "no visitors for you today?"

"Oh, I don't get visitors," Greg smiled sadly, "all my people live on the east coast."

"Well, pull up a plot of grass and enjoy the view," I said, moving to make room on the only grassy spot at the top of my hill.

"What-cha doing?"

"See if you recognize this voice," I started the recorder, over and over again.

"That's Jesse," Greg blurted, after the fifth playing.

"Jesse who?"

"Jesse Hancock," Greg repeated, "yeah.... that's Jesse all-right, he runs with William Dyse, they got busted together, William is Cuttino's cousin or something."

"What can you tell me about these two?"

"Nothing," Greg said, clearing the insensitiveness from his voice, "I don't know them to good, I just see them around... where you going?"

"Sorry Good Buddy," I said, gathering up the recorder and my notes, "I've got work to do, enjoy my hill."

"Can I come?"

"Yes," I said, clearing my thoughts, "no, on second thought, I need you here. Let me know everything you see Cuttino, Jessie and William Dyse doing. Remember Greg ... no one is to know what we are doing, do you understand that? Our lives are at stake."

"Got-cha Chief," ... my young sidekick said and rendered me a Navy salute.

The sun had risen higher in the cloudless sky as I made my way across camp to the director's office.

The visitors' parking lot overflowed, as did the kids in the visitors' picnic area.

Families huddled around tables covered with Sunday dinners. The familiar aromas took my thoughts back to the small town of Portsmouth, Virginia, and the Sunday feasts in the lot behind Saint Mark's Baptist Church.

"Mr. Chips, come meet my family," Eric Diaz called, holding up a tamale.

"Hi Diaz family," I called from the fence line, "nice meeting you, I can't come any further without an official visitor."

A tall pretty woman ran over to the fence and handed me a tamale, she was the first woman I had been close to in months. She smelled good, well, as good as I can remember a woman smelling. She was large, big breasted, big hips, big bones, and a very pretty face. I thanked her with a hug and a kiss to the cheek.

"You know you have the day off," Lloyd P. Martin said when I entered the building.

"Listen to this," I said, playing the recording of Dr. Sciortino's conversation with….

"I recognize the receiving voice," Lloyd said, moving closer to the recorder.

"Who would you say it is?" I asked, playing the tape again.

"Hancock," Lloyd said, "Jessie Hancock … What the heck is he doing in here on the phone at that hour?"

"Someone must be letting him in," I stated the obvious.

"I'll get to the bottom of this," Lloyd said, checking the duty roster.

"Lloyd, I need you to let it ride a little longer. Dr. Sciortino has something going on and the only way we can find out what it is, is to let them talk and we listen. I'll keep recording until we have something to go on. This is nothing here, but it can be our ace in the hole." I held up the recorder, "We need more, lots more."

"Well, in that case you might as well use this."

Lloyd handed me a gray metal case marked Recording Set #3.

"Oh my God, the MS-4861 listener, what are you doing with one of these?"

The MS-4861 is **the** state of the art bugging device on the market today. I'd worked with this unit once on a stakeout with the Treasury Department. —– the SDPD couldn't afford one.

I pulled the files on Cuttino Moreau, Jessie Hancock, and William Dyse, and studied them for hours.

William Dyse is indeed first cousin to Franklin Bethel Dyse, aka Cuttino Moreau. Franklin did a name change on 11-03-71, the only member of his family to turn Muslim, busted four times with first cousin William … all small stuff, possession, under the influence, disturbing the peace.

William did get popped for a 211 – robbery, never went to court, victim refused to press charges. Now, my boy Jessie is another story, converted to Islam four years ago but chose to keep his slave name, only two convictions, did seven years on a manslaughter charge. On the streets less than six months and he pops a cap in his brother's ass. His attorney pleaded it down to an assault - - - William had to give up three years.

"Lloyd, I need a big favor," I said, standing at the director's door. "Could you run these guys for me?" I handed Lloyd a piece of paper with the names of my three subjects.

"Oh Yeah …" I added, "run Dr. Sciortino, I've got to tie these four guys together."

Without questioning my reason, Lloyd took the paper and immediately made a phone call. This is the man who didn't want me in his camp, and now he had become my only comrade.

Lloyd P. Martin is a rebel waiting to explode. "Those sons-of-bitches," Lloyd cursed, "gonna use my camp to play their under-handed games and expecting me to just ride along with it."

I could be wrong, but I trust Lloyd P. Martin.

The next phone call from the Men's Colony came on Wednesday night.

The new MS-4861 recorder was programmed to record a given incoming number to a remote receiver.

Dr. Sciortino: *"My source tells me no such item was found, what's going on with you?*

Jessie: *"I put it there Doc, I swear I did."*

Dr. Sciortino: *"That was your last chance Jessie, I can't trust you."*

Jessie: *"I know, I know…. I can be trusted, give me two days Doc, I'LL THINK OF SOMETHING."*

Dr. Sciortino: *"No, I don't want you thinking. You do only what I tell you to do. Sit tight and do nothing until I tell you to.*

Jessie: *"Ok Doc, I'll wait 'til………….."*

The dial tone came in the middle of Jessie's whining.

I played the tape ten – fifteen times, nothing! It made no sense. Dr. Sciortino is up to something, I just can't see it.

Chapter – 11

FIRE

From 1945 to present, the Conservation Camp Program experienced times of expansion and decline. By 1960 … 24 - camps were in operation, 18 - camps were operated jointly between the CDF and CDC with an additional six operated in cooperation with CYA (California Youth Authority). Of the six camps operated with CYA, three were permanent and three were spike camps or temporary tent camps set up during fire season.

"FF-1 ROLLING," called the voice over the PA system, "FF-2 STAND TALL."

Firefighting team one, rolling to a two-alarm brush fire, packed up and departed camp just before lunch. FF-2 was saddled up and standing down in reserve.

"I'm one short," said Brad Duncan, lead man and youngest CDF Officer in the system.

"I'll go," I volunteered, wanting to experience a little field action, "I've been training with Team – 3."

"Watch your back out there Herman," Lloyd said, stamping my time card, "you'll be on your own."

"What's new?" I said, rushing from the office and noting the smile on Lloyd's face.

"FF-2 ROLLING," said the PA system .. and we were on the road.

Two big-yellow cattle trucks with porthole-type windows headed north from camp. It was my first rollout, and I was enjoying the adrenalin rush.

Approximately 42 miles from camp, southeast of Highway 8, just two miles south of Buckman Springs, a roaring inferno was moving to threaten the city of Jalapeno, and one of California's largest poultry farms. Six hundred and fifty-some employees worked to save 55,000+ chickens earmarked for local fast food restaurants.

Team one was clearing brush and cutting a fire line along the west perimeter. Two teams, from the CYA camps, were battling flames along the south perimeter. Team two was placed along the east perimeter, tying in with the CYA teams.

"Wiggins," called Brad Duncan, "take your squad to the top of that knoll," he pointed, "work your way west and secure Bovine Road."

Mike Balentine is the designated squad leader, who's answering questions before a child support judge ... about right now.

"Eddie," I shouted above the clamoring flames, "who's that next to you?"

"Armstrong," he answered, **working his McLeod**.

"Take Armstrong and cut an angle to your left," I ordered. "Watch your right flank, those flames are moving fast."

"Hey Sarge, I have movement on our right flank," *Corporal Finn informed, and sent his point man to recon.*

"Robbie, move your team up," I radioed, "I think we have VC activity at your one-o'clock."

"Roger – that, got 'em spotted," Robbie called back.

Motioning palms down, then a closed fist, the two Marine Recon Teams held their positions and waited. Three silent minutes later Robbie reported, "flank all-clear .... four NVA neutralized."

VC....NVA.... Wall of Fire. The enemy has to be neutralized.

1647 hours, the all-clear alarm sounded and all teams retreated to the staging area. As in combat, we were inundated with war stories, each man trying to top his neighbor.

"That was a hot one," a young man on the CYA team said to Eddie.

"You guys got your shit together," Eddie said to the young man, "how long you been doing this?"

"This is my third year on the team."

"You doing a three-year sentence?"

"With a little break in between," the young man explained, "I get released this coming Sunday."

"You stay clean brother," Eddie said, and the two men embraced, as men do in combat, after a heated battle.

"Wiggins," Lloyd called as I exited the big yellow cattle truck, I followed him to the office where two men in suits met me at the door.

"Keep your hands in view," said the first man in a dark suit, "empty your pockets and sit there."

"What's this all about," I asked, removing the last item from my coat pocket.

"Now sit down, we're asking the questions," said the second man in a light suit.

"You recognize this?" Asked dark-suit, slamming a Marine NCO Coin on the table in front of me.

"Yeah," I said, inspecting the coin, "it's my Gunny-Slug, where'd you get it?"

"How do you know Howard Newton?" Asked dark-suit.

"I arrested him numerous times."

"The records show Newton was doing time behind your arrest," said light suit.

"That's right …. I assume you guys are cops?"

"These are investigators from the Justice Department," Lloyd said, bringing me a cup of coffee, only to have it removed by dark suit.

"Mr. Martin … may we talk with Wiggins alone?" Asked dark suit.

"No, you may not," Lloyd answered, his voice charged with energy, "this is my camp and I give the final orders around here."

The suits were at a loss for words as they looked at each other in disbelief, but they knew Lloyd P. Martin was the general of this command and they needed his cooperation.

Dark suit replaced the cup of coffee and both men took a seat, settling the tension that had tightened this meeting.

"Ok Gentlemen, tell Wiggins where you're going with this," Lloyd said, taking the chair at the table across from me.

"This was found in the stream next to Howard Newton's body," dark suit said, "can you tell us how it got there?"

"I dropped it there, I swear I did," the voice of Jessie Hancock replayed in my memory and the recorded phone call was now becoming comprehensible.

"I have something I want you to hear," I said, removing the crude recorder from my desk drawer. I played the tape of Jessie Hancock and Dr. Sciortino's recorded phone conversation, identifying the two voices.

"I didn't know what this meant until now," I said, with a renewed gusto.

"My ace in the hole," Lloyd and I locked stares, laughed, and high-fived.

"Do you know who I am," I asked the two officers.

"Yeah, we heard you got railroaded," said light suit.

"Mr. Martin tells us you've been working the 187s from the inside," said dark suit.

"I hope we aren't using those words .... *from the inside*?" I looked at Lloyd, he grinned and shrugged his shoulders.

"I haven't gotten anywhere at all," I stated, "this Dr. Sciortino is doing boo-coo time at the Men's Colony. He was the BBMFIC with the San Diego Chapter of the Black Panthers when I worked undercover. My investigation sent him away for racketeering. ***From the grave, this guy is trying to frame me with these murders."***

"When you arrested Uncle Tomiko, it seems, that brought down a couple more family dominoes," Lloyd interrupted, reading from a stack of papers. "You really know how to piss-off people, don't you," Lloyd added looking at me.

"The good Doctor's wife and her family took the Doctor's estate to court and cleaned house. Mrs. Doctor is no-where to be found. The good Doctor's son was arrested for trafficking; daddy's money was keeping Junior's head above water. When Mommy Dearest cleaned house, Junior lost his grip and became a liability to his stockholders. So they gave him up to the Feds. Junior drew a 15 to 25 year stretch at Lompoc."

"Where you getting all this?" I tried to look at the papers Lloyd was reading from.

However, he moved the papers and continued, "The Doctor is uncle to his two sisters' sons, Cuttino and William Dyse, Jessie Hancock was one of the Black Panthers you busted."

"I don't remember him," I said.

"You wouldn't, he was small fry," Lloyd said. "We can't prove any of this, but we think the murders are part of a plot to frame Herman."

"These recordings are illegal and not admissible in court, you know," said dark suit.

"Thank-You-Very-Much," Lloyd and I chorused – and laughed at the insult to our education.

"We'll get a court order to tap your phones and the one at the Men's Colony," said light suit, catching our sarcasm. "Either of you have any thoughts on the murder?"

"Give us a couple of days," Lloyd said looking at me. "We might have something for you then."

We made copies of the tapes and our findings in the 187s, and sent the suits packing.

"What do we have?" I asked, watching the director break free of his cocoon and begin to enjoy his job for the first time in a long time.

Chapter – 12

TOWN MEETING

"OK – pipe down everybody, we only have the hall for an hour. I know, an hour may sound like a long time to be cooped-up in here, but believe me, an hour is not going to be enough," I said, attempting to get control of this town meeting.

"We, as a family, have been bombarded with a high degree of pressure from both the media and police investigators. Oh yeah, by the way, Willie, you sure looked good on Channels – 4 and 6."

"Hey…don't tell that ass-hole that, he don't need no mo' pumping up," said a voice from the group.

Willie…. William Hernandez – pretty boy, did some modeling, dancing, and a wanna-be actor. He had a few good recognizable walk-on parts, but in here, he's the bitch-property of Louis Rodriguez.

"OK, to start with, who has court this week?" I asked, "Willie … okay, anybody else? Mr. Ramirez also … okay…. you and me after lunch tomorrow, and Willie, you're mine tomorrow night."

"Ooooohs," murmured the group, pointing out my slip of the tongue & PC.

"Knock-it-off, we've got to work on both of you guys' testimony, don't want you representing this camp sounding like a couple of carnival workers."

"Carnival workers?" Willie asked.

"Yeah, carnival workers, you know, skinny – long shaggy hair – one tooth – with a hat size and IQ to match."

"Mr. Chips," Joel Lopez raised his hand, "have you heard anything about these murders?"

"Yeah, they're dead," another voice explained.

"Mr. Martin hasn't left any papers laying around lately," I said, reaching across the table for a cigarette from the pack sitting in front of Jessie Hancock.

"Two G-men from the Justice Department came in Tuesday, they were talking to Martin about some coin they found."

I avoided eye contact with Jessie, I just wanted to plant a little seed – and — see what grows.

"I'll do a little snooping around tomorrow morning before Martin gets in," I said. "How's everybody dealing with this murder thing?"

"I just think it's exciting," Willie said in his usual sweet-cake manner.

"Louis keep your Bitch quiet," another voice said.

"No…. no, this could be an exciting event in our lives," I said, thinking how death had made a couple of visits to our camp - and what lesson could be taught from this. "We have a killer in our midst … this community has a killer running around. Now, I don't know what we can do, but maybe … just maybe, each of us may know bits and pieces: like a puzzle."

I didn't push the **information gathering** any further. If someone had anything, the seed would pull their part of the puzzle to the table.

The in-mates were handling things fairly well, considering the little news they had received about the biggest event to ever take place at their camp.

"Mr. Chips," Ernie Leonard was waving his hand, "I got a question."

"Yes ... Mr. Leonard, what's your question?"

Ernie was a California beach boy, not the rock-group type, but a high-ranking surfer. Too much white stuff up the nose - turned him into a *space cadet*. Ernie grew up on the beach, surfing, diving, and playing beach volleyball...not an environment totally conducive to meeting a lot of Black-folks. But, he did have black friends in school, and on his father's construction crew, where Ernie worked just enough to support his surfing and cocaine passion. Doing his second stretch for possession, the color of Ernie's skin has forced him to align himself with the likes of Fred Mitchell and the Aryan Nation.

"What's-up-my-Nigga," said Ernie, his voice quivered but yet unyielding.

"Oh-No-He-Didn't," came the words from the Black side of the room.

"Oh-Yes-He-Did," I said quickly, "and I'm sure Mr. Leonard has a point."

"Yes I do ... and that's the point," Ernie's voice now stronger. "Black people don't like being called Niggers, just like White-folks don't like being called Honkies and Crackers, and I'm sure Spanish people don't want to be referred to as Spicks and Wet-backs."

"What's your point White-boy?" The words came from the Brown side of the house.

"You guys don't call yourselves Wet-backs when referring to one another, and we don't, out of respect for one another, call each other Honkies. My question is, why do Black people find the word Nigger so repulsive but constantly refer to one another as Niggers?"

First came applauds from the Brown side of the house ... soon spilling over to the White side. The Blacks sat lost for words. I didn't feel a mounting tension, just sadness at the sound of the truth.

I purposely let the applauds continue, hoping for an intelligent debate to materialize.

Ernie Leonard had stated his point so impressively … and so accurate that it could only be thought provoking.

The applauds ended leaving an uncanny feeling in the room. Both the Brown and White sides of the house thought, "how would I answer that question."

"I've always hated that *word,* even when used by other Blacks," I said, wanting to put something in the emptiness. "I've never thought of it as a term of endearment."

One by one, first the Black side of the room, then the White and then the Brown side: heads nodded in agreement, and once again, life was back to normal at Camp Rancho del Rasa.

"I also want to know why you guys gotta have your own Miss Black America" Ernie added.

"Cause you White-folks ain't got no Black women."

The room was in thought, contemplating what Cuttino had said. I wasn't sure if I understood either, but I started to applaud and everyone .. nearly everyone, joined in.

"That we will have to save for another time," I said pointing at Ernie, "see what I mean about the time flying, we are now ten minutes over our allotted time."

I looked at my watch: "Put your chairs back under the tables and get-the-hell-out-of-here, see you back at the dorm. Cuttino, give me a hand with this table?"

The camp's state of mind was going through a painful evolutionary change. Cultural sensitivity was evident, racial stereotyping was lessening, and the colors in the room were fading to neutral. This was most noticeable in the mess hall.

It was not uncommon to see a table with Blacks, Whites, and Browns eating together. Just ninety days ago such was unthinkable.

"That was a good answer you gave tonight," I said, as Cuttino Moreau and I walked to the office to turn in the key.

"Did you understand what I meant?" Cuttino asked.

"No," I answered, waiting for his response.

"Come-on Mr. Chips," Cuttino shouted, "I was hoping you'd understand," then at a lower tone, almost whispering, he said, "I was hoping you could tell me what I meant."

We both laughed … and enjoyed the cool California night.

Chapter – 13

THE HIDEWAY

By 1974, the Conservation Camp Program had changed quite a bit —- the number of camps had grown to thirty-five. Five camps were operated jointly with CYA; twenty camps were operated by CDC and CYA personnel; twenty-five camps were operated by CDF and the San Diego County Correction Department; and six Ecology Centers, where inmates with money were sent to enjoy a life of luxury.

"Yeah, Doc, it's me here," Jessie Hancock's voice came through clear on the latest recorded phone conversation.

"I understand the Feds found the coin," said Dr. Sciortino.

"Yep… just like I told you, I put it there," Jessie said.

"Ok – Ok – I heard you, now shut the fuck-up and listen. The authorities should be contacting him any day now … put the other things in his locker no later than noon tomorrow."

"How am I gonna get in his locker?"

"Parker has a master key, he'll give you a time window in which to operate."

"A what – window?"

"Just see Parker, you nitwit," Sciortino said impatiently.

"See Parker.. Gotcha Doc," Jessie answered - to a dead phone.

Some good shit, I thought, not having a plan past this moment.

I hope the Feds heard all of this back at their place, and now I've heard and know everything they know.

"Lloyd, listen to this," I played the recording, "How can I get a picture of my locker?"

"Show me where your locker's located," Lloyd said, pulling a bed assignment chart from beneath his desk blotter.

"Right here," I pointed.

"This panel ... right - here comes out," Lloyd drew a red circle around an acoustic ceiling panel directly above my bunk and locker.

"This area, all across here is reinforced, you can walk from here to your bunk.

If you lie here you can have a clear shot with a camera."

Fortunately the weather was still cool and a stakeout in the attic wouldn't be unbearable.

1000 hours: Guard Billie Parker entered the south door of the dormitory. He walked in and inspected the reading room, shower and toilet, TV room, and smoking area. He walked to the foot of my bunk, stopped and looked around 360° ... then, quickly unlocked my locker with a master key .. and slowly strolled out the north door at 1020 hrs.

I was using the new Creeper-Peeper video outfit. Lloyd, a gadget geek, buys up the latest surveillance and listening equipment as soon as it hits the market.

Some type of want-a-be super spy.

1115 hours: Jessie Hancock entered the south door of the dormitory and quickly walked to the foot of my bunk, stopped and looked to his left only. He removed a brown paper bag from his coat pocket and placed it in the bottom drawer of my locker, closed the door and relocked the locker.

"How can I see what I've got?" I asked, entering the director's office.

Lloyd pulled out another large box containing what looks like a small TV set painted a jungle-green camouflage.

"Hand me that red cable," Lloyd said, and connected it to the back of what he called an oscilloscope.

There it was, everything I needed to checkmate Dr. Tomiko Sciortino, all in living black and white.

"Parker, that SOB, I never trusted that … man," Lloyd said.

"Say it Lloyd **… that son-of-a-bitch,** it'll make you feel better, say it."

"Son-of-a-Bitch, son-of-a-bitch," Lloyd repeated, and the phone rang.

"I'll be here 'til eight," Lloyd said into the receiver, "see you at six … no thanks,

I don't eat donuts."

"I eat donuts," I whispered.

"That was Special Agent Crossland. He and his partner are about an hour away, and they have the latest phone conversation."

"I see you didn't mention the video."

"I'm saving that for when they get here. I want to see the looks on their *city boy* faces."

The special agents arrived a little before 1800 hours and came directly to the director's office, both were wearing white shirts, black ties and suits, one dark and one light, only this time they had switched.

Dark suit was identified as Special Agent Dick Crossland, and light suit identified as Special Agent Dick Kenny …… Dick and Dick.

I like the way these Fed guys say, "**Special Agent.**"

Dick and Dick were a study in contrast. Dick-C was well dressed, close cropped haircut and extremely anal in his sense of organization - a real uptight Dick.

On the other hand, Dick-K was unkempt, in bad need of a haircut. The light brown tie he wore was rumpled and stained, and his shoes were untied.

He showed no sense of organization. But Dick-K was an all around nice guy, the type you would play golf with, or go out to a ball game with.

"This is what we have," Agent Dick - C said, opening his neat briefcase and removing a small tape recorder.

"Yeah, Doc, it's me here," played the voice of Jessie Hancock in his latest prep talk with Dr. Sciortino, the same we had recorded.

"Whose locker … that's the question we need to get answered," Crossland said.

"What?" Lloyd and I said at the same time.

"What Dick here is trying to say, in his own unique way…if I may add," Dick-K took the ball, patting Dick - C on the arm, "We are here to serve a search warrant on your locker. With what we have here," Kenny patted the recorder, "it's a mere formality, keeping all of the little ducks in a row. You know how the system works."

"Then you might find this interesting," I said pressing the play button on Lloyd's super spy machine.

The small screen had our two agents at awes, but not speechless.

"How did you get this? This can't be used in court," Crossland shouted, jumping to his feet.

"Calm-down Dick," Kenny said, putting Junior back in his chair and massaging his shoulders as he stood behind him. "What we have here is not evidence, what we have here is...." Kenny stopped and pointed at me.

"An arm twister," I said. "What we have here is a people pleaser. When we sit the guilty people down in front of this tape, they will be pleased to tell us everything they know."

Flanked by the two Dicks, I followed Lloyd P. Martin to the dormitory. The other inmates were lounging in the area, but soon snapped-to when we entered the south door.

Using a master key, Lloyd opened my locker while Crossland conducted the search. Following Kenny's directions, Crossland started at the top of the locker and worked his way down to the find.

"I think we've hit pay dirt," Crossland said, emptying the contents of the brown bag on my bunk. Kenny examined the items and replaced them in the brown paper bag.

"That went well," Lloyd said, once back at the office.

"I suggest we wait about an hour .. then call Billie Parker and Hancock in to view the tapes together," I said. "Then take them to separate rooms for interrogation."

"I think we know how to handle this," Crossland said, hanging the coat of his $300 suit in the closet.

"Ok Super-Cop, how would *you* approach this," Kenny asked Crossland.

"Well ...I would ..." Crossland searched his academy memories for a solution different from mine, "the plan he said sounds good enough."

"The plan who said?" Kenny pressed.

"Wiggins' plan," Crossland shouted, and did not bother to look up.

Chapter – 14

THE TRUTH WILL SET YOU FREE

San Diego is the eloquent blend of old-world flavor and the new-age image, from its ever-growing skyline to its mega city hustle and bustle, to its luminous, almost figment beach line. And there, every evening you can watch the sun set on the horizon.

But on Monday evening, 1710 hours, San Diego Police Patrolman Richard Yescar parked his patrol car at the foot of Avenida de la Playa, as he did every evening, to watch the setting sun.

Richard works the P-2 shift … along the pacific coast .. in the community of La Jolla. He loves his job and feels that the gods are looking-out for him and only him. Why? Because of all the 15,526,891 police beats across the country, his is the best —- *La Jolla, California*.

Last week he handled six radio calls, six all week: 3 - barking dog calls,

1- leaking sprinkler, and 2 - loud music calls. "*Nothing ever happens on my beat,*" Richard thought, while he unpacked the nutritional lunch his wife of eight months insisted he eat. He got his clipboard and notes out to construct his first report of the evening, but keeping an eye on the sunset, peeping just below the upper loop of the steering wheel.

Three other cars were parked at the street bumper. As a good police officer should do, Richard checked out the two cars to his left, a single viewer on the far end, and closest to him - a young couple. On his right, there was a single viewer. All were here for the beautiful sunset.

Richard tasted the cottage cheese mixed with applesauce, *"not bad"*, he thought, although he would rather be munching on a Big-Mac right about now. *"The single viewer on his right must be sleeping,"* Richard thought, *"he hadn't moved in twenty minutes and the sun was now setting on the horizon. Should I wake him up? I would want someone to wake me."*

"There are only so many sunsets in a person's life, some people never see a PC-Sunset" his father would say, at that very spot, before he had to go off to that awful war in Vietnam… and never came home.

Richard rolled his passenger window down and called to the single viewer, trying not to disturb the other viewers. There was no response.

The sun was straddling the line.

"You're missing it," Richard shouted louder, still no response.

"Look . . . Kilroy is watching," his father would point at the quarter sun remaining.

Richard, the good-cop that he is, approached the vehicle to his right, and tapped on the window. Still no response.

"Are you okay Sir?" Richard shouted and tapped the window even harder.

Still no movement.

"Oh my God…Mother of Jesus," Richard opened the driver's door … the body of a well-dressed man fell to the ground. His raw, bloody head … which looked like it had exploded, landed on Richards's upper right leg, about crotch high, dragging bone, brains, and lots of blood down the front of his light-khaki uniform.

Richard had been a lifeguard for years but had never seen a dead body; surely he'd never touched one, and never - ever expected a mangled head to roll down his leg, soaking his uniform with blood. He could feel the blood sticking to his stomach, his legs, and his crotch.

"Unit – 12 – Unit – 12, need a supervisor at the foot of Avenida de la Playa… Code 2," Richard shouted at the police radio. "*What the fuck do I do now*," he thought, remembering he's a trained police officer with an SOP to guide his actions.

Richard contacted the people in the other cars and ascertained their vital info to give to the homicide investigators.

CSI was the first to arrive and sealed off the crime scene while Richard drowned his shaking in more hot – black - coffee.

"Suicide," said a CSI officer to the arriving homicide detectives, ".38 snub-nose in the mouth…took out all the gray matter."

2130 – hours…. ***"Just moments ago, the body of Attorney Alfonso Payton, chief aid to Superior Court Judge Green, was discovered in his car at La Jolla Cove. It appears the well known Law Review author committed suicide by shooting himself in the head"*** played the evening news on the TV in the day room at the Central California Women's Facility in Chowchilla.

"WAKE UP - WAKE UP, you gotta see this," an inmate shakes the shoulders of Angel Quick, "girl…I think we know this-here guy."

"Where are my glasses?" Angel asked, finding them on her head, "Is that who I think it is? Hand me that phone, hand me that fucking phone…now!"

"Billie, come in," Lloyd greeted the guard at the office door, extending his hand and guiding Billie to a folding chair at one end of the table.

Herman P. Wiggins, Jr.

"This is Special Agent Crossland and Special Agent Kenny."

I sat in the shadows.. and Lloyd didn't trouble to introduce me.

"Thank you for coming in Mr...." Crossland started, having to stop and read the guard's name, "Parker, Billie Parker.... is it?"

"Yes, that's it," Billie moved his big body around in the chair, trying to get comfortable.

"Is Billie a short name for William?" Kenny asked.

"No, Billie is for Billie," he said, still squirming in his chair.

"Over here Jessie," Lloyd met the inmate at the door and directed him to a folding chair next to Billie. Billie showed no change of expression ... the same lump-on-a-log look was still there.

Jessie, on the other hand, flinched. No...that black man turned pale, but the look on his face read: ***Turn-and-Run.***

"Mr. Hancock?" said Crossland.

"Jessie, Jessie will be enough, everybody calls me Jessie."

Jessie is a 26-year old kid with a 12-year old mentality, the type who needs orders and guidance.

"Jessie, I was just getting started here with Billie, you know Billie don't you?" Crossland continued.

"What's this about?" Jessie started to cry, "What he been telling you?"

"Just a minute," Crossland stepped in, "before we can move on, let's get a few formalities out of the way. We will

72

be taping this meeting and your voice will be identified on the tape."

Crossland moved a few papers around and found the one he was looking for.

"Okay, you have the right to remain silent, anything you say…" Crossland read the Miranda statement slowly.

"What's this got to do with me?" Tears ran down Jessie's face like a waterfall, he sniffed and slung snot, "I didn't do nothing."

"I just want the two of you to sit here and listen to something," Kenny said, pressing the **Play** button on the tape player.

"Doctor, it's me here, I dropped the coin where you told me to, I swear I did," the recorder played, and Jessie shook and cried even more.

Billie's expression was still unchanged.

"I don't know nothing about this," Jessie stood, shaking and pointing at the recorder, "I know, I know, I know that sounds like me, but that ain't me, he just sounds like me."

"Okay Jessie, calm down," Kenny helped Jessie back to his seat. "How you holding up over there Billie?"

"I'm here," Billie hummed his words … rocking back and forth.

"We have one more thing," Crossland regained control of the room, "watch this screen."

Kenny pressed the **Play** on the machine and the movie began, showing Billie checking out the dorm and unlocking my locker. Then … Jessie is shown entering the dorm and putting a brown paper bag in my locker … and leaving.

"On your feet…hands behind your back," the mood of the room quickly changed, "You, on the floor…don't move,"

Crossland shouted, with revolver drawn and pointed at Billie, then at Jessie.

Jessie cried louder and wanted to talk.

"Shut-up," Crossland ordered.

Jessie and Billie were handcuffed. Billie was moved to a room at the other end of the building where he was ordered to sit quietly.

Jessie talked … and talked .. and talked. One hour later, Crossland had to stop him and change the tape.

"Billie, how you feeling?" Dick-K asked, entering the room, seeing Billie resting his head on the table. "Can I get you anything?"

There was no response, as there had not been much of a response from the big fellow all night.

"Billie I want you to listen to what Jessie has been telling us, then you can make your response," again, there was no sound or movement.

Kenny pressed the **Play** button.

Jessie was heard crying, talking, and talking, and talking, and sniffing snot and tears.

"Are you listening to this?" Kenny asked, pressing the **Stop** button, "Billie you sleep?"

Kenny pushed Billie's shoulder and the big guard tumbled to the floor, lifeless. "He's dead," I said, checking his carotid artery for a pulse.

Chapter – 15

CONSPIRACY

"Can I get everyone together over here?"

2300-hours.

"Things have been developing so fast around camp today, I haven't had time to keep you guys updated."

I waited until everyone came from the shower and game room.

"Looks like some deep shit to me," Peter said.

"Who those guys searched your locker?" Billy Joe Cardoza asked, having trouble with his English.

"They were special agents from the Justice Department," I stood on my footlocker. "The Justice Department and the crime scene investigators found a special coin next to Newton's body. That coin belongs to me. The Justice Department also received an anonymous call … informing them that I was the one responsible for the death of both Zaniarripa and Newton, and that incriminating evidence could be found in my locker."

"And the Feds bought that line?" Louis Rodriguez asked, "That's about the lamest set-up I've ever heard."

"Where's Jessie?" Cuttino asked.

"Well, that's where the story moves sideways," I continued, "According to Jessie, he was working for this doctor, who's doing time at the Men's Colony, to frame me for the murders. I arrested this doctor a couple of years ago for racketeering."

"Talking about carrying a grudge," a voice chimed.

"What was the meat-wagon doing up at the office?" Curtis asked.

"Yeah, we saw them taking out a body. Didn't we Mike?" said Smiley, "We was spying from the roof."

"According to Jessie," I continued, "Billy Parker was their inside man, Billy did the killings."

"I don't believe it," Cuttino said very loudly.

The dorm was silent..........

"I would know if Jessie was involved in something this big, wouldn't I Bill?" Cuttino turns to his cousin William Dyse, "He would talk. He didn't say a word to me, he say anything to you Bill?"

Bill's answer didn't come as fast as Cuttino expected, in fact, the answer Cuttino expected never came.

"You knew?" Cuttino said, reading the blank look on Dyse's face. "You knew and said nothing to me?"

"I just found out two days ago, I swear I did, I wanted to tell you, I wanted to tell you Mr. Chips, but...Jessie, Jessie and me go way back . . . he's my homeboy."

"Bill.... you and me," Cuttino shouted, holding his cousin, "you know you can always tell me anything."

"Jessie got in some deep shit with Uncle Tommy," Dyse cried. "He said Uncle Tommy could have his legs broken if we talked."

"Uncle Tommy wants....," Cuttino said, and thought, and looked at me.

I nodded and said, "Doctor Tomika Sciortino, your Uncle Tommy, wants me dead."

The dormitory was dead silent. Dyse and Cuttino embraced, and everyone else stood frozen with shock.

"The body the EMTs took out was that of Mr. Parker," I added. "When confronted with all the evidence, we think he had a heart attack."

"Mr. Parker...dead?" someone asked.

"That's all I have now," I announced, "lights out in twenty minutes."

The dorm came alive again. Jessie Hancock's removal, and the death of Billy Parker, was like taking a handful of sand from the beach. No one cared, no one gave a rat's dump. Just another lump-of-shit hitting the fan.

"You got a letter here from the Mayor's office," Lloyd handed me a brown business size envelope, "you got connections in the Mayor's office?" I opened the envelope and read the short and to-the-point letter.

"Apparently not," I finally said, "I worked to put that SOB in office..."

"Go on, say it.... son-of-a-bitch, it'll make you feel better," Lloyd said.

"That son-of-a-bitch," I smiled, "can't afford to involve the mayor's office in my little dilemma. Godspeed ... fuck him."

"How's the morale in camp?" Lloyd asked, handing me a cup of coffee, "Here...calm down."

"The morale is great. They took all of two minutes to mourn," I said, adding more cream and sugar, "all's back to the SOS. I've got a town meeting tonight."

"You do? I didn't see a form D-61 come across my desk."

"You and your fucking forms ... Why don't you do something daring....like.... setting fire to all those forms," I pointed to the half wall of pigeonholes and neatly stacked white, and red, and yellow, and blue forms.

"We need records, we can't function without forms and records," Lloyd said seriously, and then smiled at the thought of my suggestion.

"We have a lunch meeting with your buddies from the Justice Department," Lloyd said, "We're meeting them at the State Building in El Cajon."

The near noon sun cast a short shadow of the tall palm trees lining Rancho del Rasa Road. Lloyd had all four windows down in the county car, adding another touch of freedom to the moment.

Special Agent Dick Crossland met us in the lobby, "Glad you could come," Crossland said in a friendly tone, as he extended his hand. "We have lunch set up in our conference room, follow me."

In the Marines we had a saying, "Swing with the Wing," referring to the good life in the Air Force. Looking at the El Cajon Federal Building, the local PDs should be saying ... "Swing with the Feds."

They had a two-story waterfall in the lobby, and a babbling brook that encircled the entire interior. The conference room was large and well lit, a full rib-free ceiling dome with Amplified Anon Cyper 04 glass that changed with the outside rays distributing light evenly to every corner of the room.

"Welcome to our world," Dick Kenny greeted.

Kenny was dressed up real good, well...as good as K-Mart could dress him.

His hair was cut, clean tie, still ruffled, but clean. His shoes were tied, and he had even cleaned the sleep from his eyes.

"Here – here .. you two sit here," Crossland said, pointing to two chairs across from a large movie screen that was lowering from the ceiling.

"Do we have a show for you?"

Five other agents joined us. Kenny introduced them as … *"other members of their investigative team."*

"Good afternoon Gentlemen, I'm Special Agent Jennifer Carney," a tall black woman, in a tight dark blue suit, walked to the podium. "I'll be briefing you for the first half of this meeting —- How's your lunch? Mr. Wiggins, looks like you have collected a string of enemies during your short career in law enforcement."

Jennifer had dark intelligent eyes, her lean athletic body moved in concert with the fabric of her suit … She spoke well with a precise commanding tone, managing an obvious presence of femininity.

"Angel Quick and Tomika Sciortino were contacted by someone from the old Doonsbury Machine. We don't know the identity of this person, more like a deep-throat type character. He's been the bridge in this little game of stupidity, and their plan was rather good, just poor human resource management."

"This person, or persons (unknown) in the Doonsbury camp knows how much Quick and Sciortino wants you dead. The camp is backing Quick and Sciortino's resources. They've done a very good job of building a firewall between themselves and the operation. Angel Quick has had Alfonso Payton's nuts in a vice for years. He's dancing at the end of her strings."

Special Agent Carney broke long enough to take a sip from the glass of orange juice on the podium. On the screen were pictures of Angel Quick and Dr. Sciortino. The pictures were clear enough to see their eyes, the uncompromising hate, the unforgiving eyes of my enemies. For the first time I felt the lingering powers of my adversaries.

"This is the suicide note police found in the typewriter at the home of Alfonso Payton. Payton, of the Payton family who owns much of Coronado, operates a big land development company. He was married, had two daughters, ages six and seven. And his wife Linda is from a prominent Texas oil family."

Agent Carney's cold – penetrating eyes stabbed at my consciousness, and just as quickly ... looked away, leaving a void.

Continuing ... she said.

"Alfonso was a regular at Angel Quick's bordello. I understand Alfonso approached you about getting into the honor camp system. Did he pick the camp?"

"No, I picked the camp," I corrected.

"You think you did," Carney corrected, "To pay off a debt to Quick, and keep the dark side of his life on the down-low, Alfonso put together and operated the entire conspiracy. It's all here in his seventeen-page suicide manuscript. Names, dates, but no strings to the Doonsbury camp. Rancho del Rasa was the perfect camp. There are more convicts there that you've arrested than at all the other camps combined. The powers-to-be hadn't counted on your survival skills. When the inmates didn't do the job, another plan had to be implemented. Sciortino got his dim-witted son...."

"Son?" Lloyd and I said together.

"Jessie Hancock is one of many of the good Doctor's kids running around Southern California, Jessie was the weak link."

Agent Carney concluded, looking down at me from behind the podium, she said, "Good luck ... watch your back ... We have the monster's body and the tail, however … the head is capable of growing another body."

"I'm Bob Butler," said the next speaker, changing places with Agent Carney.

"Special Agent Bob Butler…" he corrected himself. Butler is young agent who has a grossly ordinary appearance, average height, average weight, and a face you would not remember an hour later, but he moved with the willingness of a man who overlooks rules.

"Special Agent Butler is one of our little geniuses around here," said a man identified as the district manager, looking at Butler with pride and undisguised respect.

"Arrest warrants were served on Angel Quick, Tomika Sciortino, and Jessie Hancock, for murder, conspiracy, and obstruction of justice," the young agent continued. "Semen found on the body of Adam Zaniarripa matches the blood type of Billy Parker, which verifies what Jessie told us. The items found in your locker: drivers license and inmate ID belonging to Zaniarripa and Newton had the fingerprints of Billy Parker and Jessie Hancock, none of yours. I wish we could say '*that's a wrap*', but that's not the case.

As Jennifer put it, the head still lives out there, we're sure they will try and make another run at you."

Getting away from camp, if only for a couple of hours or so, was a breath of fresh air. As we drove back that afternoon, I knew, absence did not make the heart grow fonder.

Chapter – 16

I DON'T CARE

June marks the beginning of fire season. Last year's heavy rainfall left California's hills and fields rich with a new growth of vegetation.

Southwest of camp, through the tall grass and desert shrubs, past the line of Joshua trees, are the ruins of the first permanent camp established in 1942, Coursegold Honor Camp.

The term **honor camp** was replaced with **conservation camp** in 1959, a term still used today.

Conservation projects, then … as now, consist of maintenance of state parks, erosion control, and the care and growth of tree seedlings at state nurseries.

Over the years, records show that four percent of the inmates passing through the system go on to study and receive degrees in forestry related subjects.

"Something to think about, Herman," Lloyd handed me an employment form,

"I could use you back here after your time's up."

"You gotta be kidding," I said, looking at the form and tossing it back to Lloyd. "When my time's up, I'm outta here."

"You have something to offer these guys. I've never met anyone with such a command presence .. You care about them, and they respect you."

"Bull-shit," I said, and left it there.

"Bull-shit, what's bull-shit, the way you feel about them or the way they feel about you?" Lloyd asked.

"Both...Lloyd, you've been in the system long enough. These guys are prime-time con artists. I have to think that way. I've got to be as big or a bigger con artist. I'm doing time... it's up to me as to what type of time I want to do, hard time or soft time. I'm the captain of my world. My life, my destiny is in my hands only. I did not come into this camp praying for God's protection. I set the tone of this camp for my survival only."

"What about all those classes and self-help lecturing you've been doing?"

"All a con .. all a game Lloyd... When I checked in here I had no idea what I was going to be facing. All I knew was that there's a whole bunch of people out there who want to kill me, and I knew I had to establish the tone at the gate. See those brochures?" I pointed at the wall display rack with 78 different booklets.

"See how dusty they are? No one reads those things ... I did ... each and every one of them. From those dusty old papers I created my character, *the teacher.*

I put together twelve lesson plans, calling them *Info-for-dummies.* Who are the most loved and respected people in a community...the *teachers*.

"You go to the teacher for knowledge and help. I've got these dick-heads eating out of my hands. It's all about surviving, Lloyd. I'm playing a part. Don't mistake my character for the real thing. I don't give a flying-fuck about these losers."

"I don't believe that," Lloyd said, giving me one of his incredulous stares.

"Believe it my friend, all I want is to do my time, like in Vietnam ... and go home with everything I came here with."

Lloyd seemed half convinced ... well, maybe that's a good sign. If my performance here is good enough to convince the director, that's half the battle.

I don't give a rat's ass about these losers, I thought of my words that night while sitting on my bunk, *I don't care, I can't afford to care.*

I looked around the dorm, Billy Joe and Ernie Leonard played a game of chess, Billy Joe knows how to write a résumé now ... he gets out this Saturday ... he's been mailing résumés out and has five bites to choose from.

Kevin Johnson is ready for the streets, we worked on his composition writing, and he's able to pass the GED test.

But my greatest pride is in Michael Molina ... he received his citizenship papers last week. We went over every question at least 50 times.

"What you doing Mr. Chips?" asked Bryan Karpov, a staunch White-Supremist,

"I never see you writing letters."

"Don't have anyone to write to, Bryan," I said. "What are you doing wandering around, no TV for you tonight?"

"Too many commercials," Bryan said, taking a seat on the bunk next to mine, "don't like commercials."

"Who does," I said, watching my guest rock back and forth ... sucking his thumb.

"You okay, Bryan?"

"Don't like commercials...commercials no-good."

"Talk to me Bryan, what are you thinking about here?" Bryan was beginning to freak me out. "Why don't you like commercials?"

Bryan started to cry. "When I was a little boy ... every time a commercial came on my mother would send me to get something ...I could never please her ... She would complain that I took too long or I brought the wrong thing and ... then, then she would beat me."

"I take it you don't like your mother?"

"I think she's dead," Bryan quickly stood, looked up at the ceiling, and sat down just as quickly.

"No, I love my mother ... she's a good Christian woman ... it was those commercials, they made her do it...they made her do things to me."

I...well...I was at a loss for words, as I watched the young man with swastikas on both biceps cry, suck his thumb, and cuddle my neighbor's pillow.

"Good morning Lloyd," I greeted the next day. "What can you tell me about Bryan Karpov?"

"He should be locked up," Lloyd said, not looking up from what he was so busy with on his desk.

"He is locked up .. Lloyd," I reminded.

"No, I mean locked up in a state hospital, Karpov is sick, I've put that in every report about his status."

"Last night he was murmuring something about his mother and TV commercials. Says his mother beat him, but he still loves her," I said, pausing to read Bryan's record book. "He did a stretch at Vacaville Psychiatric State Hospital?" I read aloud. "He loved his mother to death," Lloyd added.

"Eighteen months in the hospital for killing his mother," I said, reading the SY-540 form in Bryan's CRB, "that's all, eighteen months?"

Now, I wonder if Bryan had been reaching out for my help last night. I didn't pick-up on it.

It was going to be a good day — the air was warmer than the day before —and the five-day forecast was saying, "*WELCOME TO SPRING*". I enjoyed the morning and its clear mountain air with a cup of jailhouse coffee and a cigarette.

"Why the long face Darren, for a man going home tomorrow, you don't look all that happy," I said.

"Going back to the same old shit," Darren said, not missing a stroke with the yard rake he used each morning to line the sand in front of the camp office.

"Trouble with the old lady on the home front?" I asked, sitting on a box watching Darren work.

Darren Arabia caught eight months for battery on his wife. His public defender lost a good self-defense case. Darren, 55, is 5'-3" and 117-pounds soaking wet; his wife, a mail-order bride from the Midway Islands is a plus size woman, 6'-3" 299-pounds. Mrs. Arabia lands in the hospital with a strained back after throwing Darren from the window of their second floor apartment; the police arrest Darren.

"Don't seem to have enough between the legs to keep the missus happy these days," Darren explained.

"Wooo … a little more information than I need," I smiled at the old fellow. "You know what they say, it ain't the size of the boat that counts, it's the motion of the ocean. You heard that .. haven't you?"

"All the motion in the ocean ain't gonna help my little dick."

"Come on Darren, can't be that small."

"Yes it is," he boasted, dropping his pants and exposing a penis about the size of a swollen clitoris.

"Okay…." I stuttered, "I think you've made your point."

"I wish I had a black dick."

"Come again?"

"Yeah, like all you black guys. If a genie gave me three wishes, one would be to have a black dick. Mr. Chips, I bet you're hung."

"No, not at all Darren, I was out surfing with the White guys when God handed out all those black dicks."

I finally got a smile out of Darren, he worked his way around the building, laughing out loud.

"Maybe I do care," I said, standing at Lloyd's office door.

"Care about what?" Lloyd asked, looking over his skinny reading glasses.

"These guys…maybe I do care. I've seen so many of them grow."

"You've helped them grow," Lloyd said leaning back in his chair, tossing his glasses and pencil on the desk. "I knew all along you cared, this is your calling."

"And who's calling me to this job?"

"I am…CAN'T YOU HEAR ME….HELP!"

And it was my time to laugh.

Chapter – 17

BIG BAD JOHN

I must admit I was beginning to feel pretty good about myself and the way I'd managed to survive eight months of incarceration. In fact, I was feeling extremely cocky when thinking of my many accomplishments at Rancho del Rasa.

That is until July 14th, Tuesday, 0945-hours. The day and hour my worst nightmare came to town. John Lee Landenberg …the biggest - and - baddest mother fucker I have ever met.

I first met John in 1970 while working the night shift out of Central. I was a rookie working Logan Heights; it was my first night in the Heights.

My partner was Tom Watson, a seasoned veteran with nine years on the streets. Tom knew everybody and everything there was to know about every street hood, hooker, and harlot.

"Units in the area of 49th Street and National Avenue: Be on the lookout for a John Lee Landenberg, male Black, wanted for the attempted murder on his girlfriend," said the dispatcher.

"My old friend Big John," Tom said, looking through a small file cabinet he carried in the back seat of the patrol cruiser.

"Here we go," Tom pulled a 4x5 card with a small booking photo of a light complexioned – male — Black. Tom read the vital-stats, placing emphasis on BIG and DANGEROUS.

"Turn right at the next street," Tom pointed, "John's mother is on the left … that brown and white house there."

I parked two houses away.

It was a typical warm July night, clear skies and lots of kids playing in the street.

"Cover the back door," Tom ordered, looking at his watch, "I'll give you one minute to get in position."

"Any dogs?" I questioned, with great concern in my voice.

"No dogs," Tom smiled, "Mom is allergic to cats and dogs."

Now, how would he know that, or even better, why would he know that?

Good, I thought, making my way through the maze of junk collected in the small backyard.

Knock-Knock-Knock, "POLICE," I could hear Tom announce our arrival. There was no response, no sound, or movement.

Tom entered the unlocked door and found John sleeping on a sofa.

"Herm, he's here," Tom called.

I entered the back door and saw Tom trying to awake a human giant.

The man sat up and ran his thick fingers through his long Jheri-curled hair.

The front of his shirt was covered with blood, as were his hands and shoes.

"John, you awake?" Tom bellowed.

"What the fuck you want?" Were the giant's first words, looking first at Tom then at me.

"John, we're here to take you downtown for slicing up your girlfriend," Tom said. "Do you understand me?"

"Did the bitch die?" He asked, rubbing his eyes with the back of his huge hands. "No, but you left her pretty fucked-up," Tom informed John.

"She should be dead, fucking bitch ... caught her going deep-throat on my main man ... fuck her," he slumped back on the over-stuffed sofa that was covered with clear plastic.

On the coffee table were three empty beer bottles, one half empty - or half full - bottle of Black Label. Five empty beer cans were lying on the floor around the sofa.

"John, we don't want any trouble," Tom said standing to John's right. I was standing to his left with handcuffs in one hand and a Cal light in the other.

"Please stand up and put your hands behind your back."

"Where's your back-up," John slurred, looking at his bloody shirt and hands for the first time.

"We're it John," Tom said. "We ... my partner and I are taking you in."

"The fuck you are," John struggled to get his big body up from the sofa; and when he did, he grew, and grew, and grew until his head nearly touched the ceiling.

This was the tallest man I had ever seen. His shoulders had to be as wide as I am tall. My nose came to his waistline.

"You and this little girl?" He laughed, his deep loud voice shook the room, "you don't want to fuck with me, do you little girl?" The giant looked down at me, and my first thought was, *"No sir, we were just joking, you go on back to sleep and act like we never disturbed you."*

"Herman," Tom shouted, snapping my attention back to real time, "remember what I told you about Big John?"

My second thought was, *"no, I don't want to remember, let's go home, and why is it we didn't call for back up, you knew how huge this mother fucker was."*

"Officer Wiggins," Tom called again, noticing how the giant's size had hypnotized me, "what did I tell you about Big John?"

Big John, 7-feet - 10-inches, 474-pounds … I mentally reviewed the big-man's rap - sheet … wrestled under the ring name of Pretty Boy John. Ooooh-yeah…. Big John's wrestling career ended with an ulcer, *a — bad — stomach - ulcer.*

Nodding to Tom, I laid the shaft of my eighteen-inch Cal light in the giant's stomach, using every bit of strength and power my .. *little girl's..* body could muster.

John's arms shot up to the ceiling. His big knuckles broke through the drywall bringing popcorn acoustic down around us like snow on a winter day in Denver.

"Oh my God," he cried, spitting a spray of blood across the room to the next wall. Then, without another sound, the giant fell … face down … across the large antique coffee table.

"You okay?" Tom asked me.

"No, I'm not okay," I shouted, "Tell me again … why didn't we call for cover?"

"For what," Tom laughed at me shaking, "all it took to bring him down was … one little girl."

And to that … I had to laugh.

My second encounter with John Landenberg was a week later at his arraignment in Municipal Court, Department – 11.

Tom and I were sitting in the front row when John was brought in and placed in a glass cage, his ankles were shackled, as were his hands to his side. His long Jheri-curled hair was matted, and the pretty boy image was gone.

John hadn't noticed Tom and I, he came in quietly and took a seat behind the glass shield.

"He doesn't look so bad now, does he," Tom said.

"The fuck he don't," I replied, not being able to take my eyes off the freak of nature. "That has got to be the biggest mother in the world."

"Watch this," Tom whispered, smiling and sticking his tongue out at John, who was now staring us down.

"You goddamn mother-fucking-pigs," John shouted, standing and banging his head on the glass shield, "I'm gonna kill you....you hear me, Goddamn Pigs, and you, yes you little girl, I'm gonna fuck you in the ass, you hear me."

I wanted to move to the other side of the room. If that glass breaks, no.... when that glass breaks, I wanted more of a head start.

John carried on for so long and was so loud ... the judge had to have him removed from the court.

And here he is, the newest inmate at Camp Rancho del Rasa.

Fuck ... just what I didn't need right about now.

"Big-son-of-a-bitch," Lloyd said as we watched the giant unfold his oversized body from the white county van.

"Big and even badder attitude," I added.

"You know this guy?"

"I sure do," I said, trying not to show fear in my voice, "I arrested him a few years ago."

"Why am I not surprised," Lloyd said, looking straight ahead, "think he'll remember you?"

"I'm sure he will, there's no doubt about it."

John had gotten even bigger than I remembered, putting on thirty to forty pounds around the mid-section.

"John Landenberg, welcome to Rancho del Rasa," Lloyd met the new inmate at the office door, "I'm the Camp Director, these are my staff members and...."

Lloyd gave Big-John his usual 30-minute welcome aboard talk, introducing the staff and reading the long list of do's and don't do's.

I sat at my desk with my back to the processing, hoping to prolong the inevitable.

Chapter – 18

THE SHOWDOWN

"Did you see that big fellow they just brought in?" Darren asked, "he looks like he eats nails for breakfast ... wouldn't want to be on his bad side."

"Me neither," I said, knowing the big showdown had to be today.

I'm not the type that's easily intimidated. Before meeting John Landenberg, I was a staunch anti-death penalty advocate. Now, I believe that there are some people who just don't deserve to live among the rest of us.

1145-hours, "FORMATION – NOON FORMATION," called the PA system.

Inmates strolled in from every corner of the camp. Each formation is mandatory, noon formation is for head count #3 and lunch.

"Officer Wiggins," John shouted, as I approached the workout field with the other inmates at Camp Rancho del Rasa, "I heard you were here, have you missed me?"

"And you are.......?" I asked.

"How could you forget me," John roared, stepping out of formation, "I have waited and dreamed about this day."

"Oh yeah... John Landenberg," I stared the giant down, trying to hide my trembling emotions.

"Remember what I told you the last time I saw you?"

"No John, I don't ... but I'm sure you have every intention of reminding me."

The formation of inmates stood by quietly … anticipating something. The smell of adrenalin thickened the air, this was surely the showdown I had dreaded and had nightmares about.

"You are going to be my bitch," John's voice was as loud and intimidating as ever, "right here, now, in front of God and everybody, I am going to fuck you in the ass."

John and I stood facing one another approximately 30 feet apart, the noon sun was directly above — John's large nose was casting an eerie shadow over his mouth. I was smiling, almost laughing, when John started walking in my direction.

"Drop your panties little-girl and grease down your asshole, or would you rather suck my dick?" the giant said, now running at me in a slow trot picking up speed with every step.

"I'm here to fulfill a promise," John shouted, telegraphing a right-hook,

I stood my ground allowing the big guy to bring the fight to me. Just as he reached the two-foot mark, I dropped to the ground and assumed a fetal position.

John's momentum brought his mid-section in contact with the heel of my right boot, thrusting upward with a one count Yo-Ti-Lee kick, stopping him long enough for me to spin right and crash the side of my left boot into the right side of his face.

The giant gasped for one last breath of air as he fell face first into the horseshoe pit.

"**Get the nurse!**," I directed the closest inmate, catching my breath and counting my loud sounding heartbeats.

It was three days later when John was released from the hospital. My report of the incident, along with the written observation of twelve inmates who were directed by Lloyd to make a statement, was forwarded to the Corrections Department.

"Mr. Landenberg, we have enough here to roll you back to county," Lloyd said, waving his copies of the investigation, "It's up to you. Herman here is not pressing charges, so what do you want to do?"

John looked tired, like the fight had drained from his veins. He stood with a slump, and the giant I feared didn't seem so ferocious any more.

"Where you learn that shit?" John asked softly.

"In the Corps," I said.

"You think you could learn me?"

"Is that what you want?"

"Yeah, you win, I'll say uncle if that's what you want."

"Uncle?" I thought out loud, "Yeah … I would like to hear you say UNCLE."

"Ok … ok … **_UNCLE_**," unenthusiastically, John's big lips formed the word.

"We have Jujitsu classes on Tuesdays and Thursdays nights, you're welcome to come." I forced a smile and extended my hand.

"You teach this stuff?"

"Yes…have for years."

"Why didn't you tell me that before I made a fool of myself out there?"

"You didn't ask."

John smiled for the first time.

"We don't expect a repeat match, do we?" Lloyd asked.

"No…. not from me," John said with a shrug."

"Good…. take your bags back to the dorm and report to the tool shed," Lloyd said.

"What about those Little-Girl remarks?" I added.

"Ain't seen no Little-Girl with a kick like that," John said, moving towards the door. "More like a little horse," he said, and limped away.

"You sure about this?" Lloyd asked, after John had left the office. "That guy's a little touched in the head."

"He's okay now," I said, praying under my breath that I was right, "He's my therapy, I'll keep him around as an example."

"Hope you know what you're doing. Oh…here…you've got a letter from the Governor's office."

"My boy Jerry," I said, opening the envelope and noticing that Governor Bendell didn't write the letter.

"The Governor is in receipt of your letter dated: 03 March," I read out-loud. *"The Governor is interested in the information you forwarded in your second letter dated 17 April. The appropriate division of the Justice Department has been notified. Governor Bendell recommended, to the County of San Diego, your immediate release to a Sober Living Program while the Justice Department completes its investigation."*

"What's a Sober Living Program?" I asked Lloyd.

"A half-way house. . . the county has these houses, mostly in the inner-city, where they house anywhere from fifteen to twenty-five inmates," Lloyd explained, "They have a cook, dining facilities, four to six men per room, and a game room with library and study hall."

"Sounds like my kind of place."

"You get to leave during the day and go to work," Lloyd added, "Have any idea where you'll work?"

"Oh yeah, Barnum Diving, the owner's a close friend."

"Rancho del Rasa," Lloyd answered the phone, "Yes…he's standing right here," Lloyd looked at me, "sure, Mr. Wiggins just received the letter."

Lloyd handed me the phone, smiling.

"Hey dickhead," the voice on the other end said.

"Hello, who's this?"

"Lewis Mitchell, done forgot me already?"

"Lewis, how the hell you been?" I now recognized my attorney's voice.

"I see you're still hob-knobbing with the brass," Lewis said, with a smiling tone. "All about surviving, my friend, what's going on?"

"You're checking into Garfunkel House on Wednesday, they hope to have a bed open by then. All hell is breaking loose downtown .. my sources tell me. Sacramento has investigators crawling all over city hall and the police station."

"What's all this have to do with me?"

"The Governor's office wants you nearby and accessible. My sources also tell me that something has come to surface that could lead to all charges in your case being dropped."

"YES! That's what it's all about," I shouted, *in a smiling tone*. "I'm back in the game again."

"Slow down there Devil Dog," I could see Lewis holding up his hand, "let the boys from Sacramento do their job. I understand there's still a price on your head."

"Still a price on your head," the words tore into my consciousness like a hot knife through butter.

The burning reality that so many people wanted me dead should have been depressing, or at the least frightening. I felt neither. The adrenalin had me high again, all I knew … *I was back in the game*.

"Can we keep this silent until tomorrow night?" I asked Lloyd.

"Secret … sure, I was going to suggest that."

I made a call to Jeffery Barnum, owner and manager of Barnum Diving.

"You got it good buddy, just at the right time too, I'm short an instructor," Jeffery was saying with a welcoming voice.

Everything was smiling in my life again, but the reality of an all-new set of problems at a half-way house hadn't yet set in. Who – and - what I would have to be to become head of household, was just another game to be played.

Tuesday – 1900-hours – Town Meeting – Camp Rancho del Rasa.

The mess hall / meeting room was brightly lit, Paul Castellano, the camp cook, was still on duty cooking up something that was smelling mighty good.

The troops were strolling in, eyeballing the table of goodies the cook's crew had put out: Six types of donuts, crumb cakes, apple – cherry – and peach pies, with cups of vanilla – strawberry – and chocolate ice cream.

In the kitchen, Paul was cooking up those pizzas he was so famous for, and took pride in. He was always talking about how his grandfather had to smuggle the recipe out of the old country.

"Everybody grab a plate of munchies and something to drink and take a seat,"

I said, putting together a plate, a big plate of heart stoppers and artery blockers.

"What's up with all the goodies?" Tom Little asked.

"Some kind of celebration, I suppose," One-Finger Henry answered.

"We have a few matters to tend to tonight," I started, "so let's get this show on the road."

"What's happening Mr. Chips?" Ernie Leonard asked.

"Yeah, what's with the party here?" Cuttino stood, pointing at the table and kitchen area.

"You're right, this is a party," I said, "we are here to celebrate the new camp Mayor."

The room quickly grew silent, a blank stare from every pair of eyes, to include Bobby Smith's single eye, was fixed on me.

"And we could say it's my going away party," I added, and the hall came alive again.

"Governor Jerry Bendell has taken an interest in Mr. Wiggins' case," Lloyd said, walking into the hall from the kitchen. "This is his last night with us."

"The Governor?" a voice called out.

"Hey Mr. Chips, turn the Governor on to me," called another voice.

The whistles and cheers came, so did the applauds.

"Mr. Chips – Mr. Chips – Mr. Chips – Mr. Chips – Mr. Chips – Mr. Chips," they chanted and stomped their feet.

"Thank you – thank you," I held both hands up, to quiet the meeting, "we still have to vote in a new mayor, any nominees?"

"What's a **nominee?** " Greg Abboud asked another inmate.

"Like a want list, I think.... I don't know!" the inmate answered.

"You tell me who you would like to see as your Mayor, and that person will be the nominee." I answered their question.

"Who would you like to put in that seat, Mr. Chips?"

I hadn't wanted this decision, although I had thought of my choice, I was hoping the question wouldn't come up.

"Okay, this is not a nomination," I said reluctantly, "I don't get a vote, but if I did, I think Mr. Rodriguez is up for the job."

Again, silence cloaked the room, I locked eyes with Louis Rodriguez, they were smiling words of thanks.

"I'll give a thumbs up to that," a voice said.

"Mr. Rodriguez got my vote," another faceless voice said.

"Me three," said another.

"I want to nominate Willie Hernandez," Fred Mitchell said.

"Sit down Freddy, all you're voting for is a head-job," a voice from the north side of the room said.

"I-beg-your-pardon," Sweet Willie took the floor, "I do more than just give head." He turned and shook his girlie shaped butt at the group.

"I nominate Louis Rodriguez," Cuttino Moreau said.

"I'll second that," Fred Mitchell said, "you the man Louie."

"Any other nominees?" I asked, looking around the room, "Ok … lets see a show of hands on this nominee."

Every hand in the house was raised … even Louis' hand.

"Well …looks like Mr. Rodriguez is our new Mayor."

All, including the camp director, congratulated Louis.

He was beaming and glowing with pride as the other inmates gathered around to give support to their new camp Mayor.

Cuttino Moreau or Fred Mitchell could have stepped up to the plate, but Louis was the best political choice … and they all knew it.

The meeting adjourned, and the inmates loaded their pockets, clearing the goodie table for a promising late night snack.

"Thanks for your vote of confidence," Louis said, extending his hand, "it has been an honor knowing you."

"Like Fred said … you the man now," I accepted his hand in both of mine.

Then they all came, one by one, extending their hands, Blacks – Whites – Browns. No color barriers existed that night. Camp Rancho del Rasa is my rainbow, they spoke from the heart, words of thanks, congratulations, and….

"You-go-get-'em Mr. Chips."

Wednesday – 0940-hours:

"Watch your back Herman," Lloyd said, walking me to the white county van, "Half-way houses have bad guys too. You don't want to get this close and take a shank in the ribs one night."

"I'll be careful," I answered, with a tear in my voice.

"It's been good working with you," Lloyd hugged me, "thanks for all your help here, think about my offer. I put the forms in your paperwork folder."

"If I ever did come back here," I said, as I climbed in the shotgun seat, "my first official act would be to set fire to that **form rack** of yours."

Lloyd laughed, took one step back, saluted, and mouthed, "good luck my friend." And the van drove through the gate and beneath the huge red and gold sign depicting the end of an adventure at Camp Rancho del Rasa.

Chapter – 19

GARFUNKEL HOUSE

Seeing the San Diego skyline for the first time in nine months brought a lump to my throat and a tear to my eye.

San Diego's natural beauty is one of its greatest attractions. I conjured up fond memories of my life in San Diego as the van drove through Balboa Park and its 1200-acres, home to the world-famous zoo and museums. The park is the cultural center of the city. The rose garden has more than 2,000 rose bushes. The entire park is one giant botanical garden of beautiful flowers and trees.

In the 1960s, with the aerospace industry in a decline, San Diego entered a down period. Time magazine carried a story in 1964 that labeled San Diego: "Best Town USA."

At the same time, seeds were being planted that would ultimately grow into San Diego's future economy. Two of those seeds took root in La Jolla … the opening of the Salk Institute … and the 1000-acre University of California at San Diego Campus.

Meanwhile, tourism began to emerge as a factor in San Diego's economy.

San Diego has it all: Sunny weather .. Great beaches .. and a fascinating history.

"Welcome to Garfunkel House Mr. Wiggins," greeted a tall - frail man with lots of graying hair. "Let me introduce myself, I'm Dwight Ackley, Director, here at Garfunkel."

Dwight's voice was strong, a touch of a British twang, but with a commanding presence, unlike his appearance.

Garfunkel House was much more than I had expected, a two-story Victorian-style home once owned by one of San Diego's wealthiest families. It was declared Historical Landmark # 224 on 21 June 1942, and purchased by the county in 1952.

"Eighty percent of the teakwood, you see lining these fifteen foot walls, is the original wood from the Continental Navy Ship, *Alfred,* placed in commission December 1775 and commanded by Capt. Dudley Saltonstall," Dwight said in one breath, while giving me the VIP tour, "There are twenty-three pieces of priceless antiques displayed throughout."

"It's like taking a walk back through history," I said, marveling at the beauty and history of the old house. "How can the county afford this place?"

"I'm also the curator of this museum," Dwight proudly informed me, ignoring my question, "only selected inmates are assigned here."

The place was immaculate ... large paintings of past U.S. Presidents hung in every room.

The Hacienda-style landscape and manicured lawns gave Garfunkel House a majestic and alluring appeal appreciated by the most discriminating palate.

Twelve extremely low security inmates were housed at Garfunkel: 3 - attorneys, 2 - politicians, 4 - business executives, 2 - actors, and me.

And me ... why me? ... How did I end up here on Knob-Hill?

"This is your room," Dwight said, unlocking a tall dark wood door and handing me the key, "your roommate is Danny Todd."

"Danny Todd?" I snapped.

"I'm sorry, is that going to be a problem? This is the only empty bed we have left. I did have a long talk with Danny and he's ok with having you here."

County Supervisor Danny Todd got caught up in the **Doonesbury** fiasco. The promising career of a small duck, in the dirty political pool, came to a screeching halt. A 32-year-old Harvard Law grad and son-in-law of oil magnum Ronald Hathaway, Danny Todd lost it all … His wife of five years packed up and moved back home to daddy, taking everything Danny had, including the love of his life, his three-year-old daughter, Sheri.

On the nightstand next to his bed was a picture of him, his wife, and daughter standing in front of what looks like a very – very nice house.

"I'll leave you to settle in," Dwight said. "The house schedule, along with all the rules and regulations are in your welcome folder. Mr. Todd gets home around five, you've got about an hour. Dinner starts at five and ends at seven."

The room was large, 30 X 30, with one of those high-beamed ceilings. A waist high dresser ran three-quarters of the room and divided it into two comfortable living spaces, it had two bathrooms and one TV.

So, this is Club Med … county style.

"The infamous Mr. Wiggins," said Danny Todd, the all-American boy, as he entered the room, "welcome to The Garfunkel Cell … that's what we call it around here. Just don't let Colonel Ackley hear you. You would think this place is his private residence. He lives here, you know, been here for over thirty years. The word is he hasn't left the place in ten years, never been married, has no lady friends…"

Danny was straight off the Wheaties box, he was tall, blonde, with an athletic body . . . even had a Clark-Kent type of jaw, and talked a-mile-a-minute.

"So, what do you think of this place?" I asked.

"Not bad, give me a minute to wash-up, we'll walk down to the dining room together. This is crazy… isn't it?"

"What's crazy?" I asked, loud enough to be heard over the running water.

"You and me .. putting you and me in the same room .. we've never met.

I've watched you on TV when you were going through your trial."

"I'm glad you're taking this the way you are."

"I've never blamed you for what happened to me," Danny said, sticking his head out the bathroom door, "I knew what was going on. I wouldn't take any money. But to save my job … I helped in the cover-up. Now I wish I had taken the money. At least I would've walked away with something."

"So this is your reward for not being a whistle blower?"

"The money wasn't worth it. From what I understand, at first it was. The Mayor and his boys were skimming off a seven-figure kickbacks. Before long, everybody and their mother had hands in the pot."

"What line of work are you in now?"

"I'm an auto mechanic," Danny said, pointing to the uniform he was shedding, "Come on, let's go dine. I love working on cars, my father was a mechanic. Between the ages of 12 and 19, my dad and I rebuilt an old 1941 Ford Super Deluxe from the ground up. I wanted to be a mechanic and Dad wanted to be a lawyer. He was the mechanic, so I guess I had to be the lawyer … you do the math."

The way to the dining hall took us through parts of the house I hadn't seen, "Isn't this unbelievable," Danny said as we walked down the long hall, much narrower than normal.

Shiny black oak planks lined the walls that extended to a height of twenty feet, illuminated red abstract paintings hung randomly along the corridor.

"Here we are," Danny opened the door to the room King Arthur and the Knights of the Round Table must have used. There was one large round table .. 20 to 25 feet in diameter.. with high-back chairs comfortably spaced. In the center of the table was a fire pit, and above that a large hood that climbed nearly 30 feet to the ceiling.

"Buffet tonight. Tuesdays, Thursdays, and Sundays is sit-down and order from menu nights. All other nights ...buffet."

Two other men were entering the dining hall about the same time, Danny did the introductions.

"I'm out of here in 35 days," Danny said, "I'm joining Olson, Menze and Kesler as a law clerk ... just long enough to get my license back. What about you?"

"Diving instructor," I answered, "teaching sport SCUBA diving over at Barnum's."

"Got any family?"

"No .. not really .. well, I have a daughter .. she's with my ex-wife. I don't know where they are."

Danny and I talked about every subject under the sun until 4:00-AM.

By the time the alarm went off, I was just shifting into second gear. The heavy burgundy drapes impeded the morning light. Except on this morning, a slight opening allowed a slither of sunlight to enter the room ... and it fell across my face.

Chapter – 20

BACK IN THE GAME

State of California Department of Justice.

The office of the Attorney General represents the people of California in civil and criminal matters before trial, Appellate and the Supreme Court of California.

The Special Investigation team from Sacramento set up operations in the old Barnna State building at 1201 Harbor Boulevard.

"Good morning Herman, I'm Mike Mattox," said the line-backer-size man, "glad you could join us. Can I get you a coffee?"

"No thanks, I'm good," I said, following Mike through the maze of desks, file cabinets, and stacks of books.

"Have a seat, I apologize for the mess. As disorganized as we may look, to that same degree we've got it together."

"What about Mr. Tyree's office downtown, isn't he working on this?"

"We're keeping his office abreast of our investigation. I understand you and his son were in the Marines together?"

"Yeah, Jack was my best friend."

"You guys keep in touch?"

"Not for a couple of years … he married some rich movie producer's daughter… Sent me a post-card from somewhere in Kazakhstan where he was shooting a movie."

"Rich producer's daughter … Yoooo," Mike smiled.

The morning sun was heating the easterly facing office, and casting a long shadow over the tuna boats preparing for an AM mooring.

"I know, we get started around here quite early, but you know what they say, *'the early bird gets the worm'*, and we do have a few worms to catch," Mike said, placing a stack of files on the desk in front of me.

"Need you to take a look at these files and make a note of everything that rings your bell."

"There has to be a week's work here," I mumbled.

"More like three weeks," Mike added two more stacks.

"What about my job at the dive shop?"

"This is your job," Mike said, adding another stack of files.

"You're on the payroll as of today."

"Working for the Attorney General's Office?"

"You-got-it," Mike handed me a contract stating my employment and salary of $1000 a month.

"You in?" Mike handed me a pin.

"I'm in … I guess," I took the pin and signed my way back into the game.

"Federal and State investigators have discovered a number of bookkeeping irregularities in their probe of the 1972 Doonsbury scandal," read Edwin Whipple, lead anchor – Channel 4 News, *"It appears that city resources were used to set up the State's largest numbers-running racket in the history of San Diego."*

"Did you know about this?" I asked Danny as we watched the 11 o'clock news.

"I'll-be-a-son-of-a-bitch," Danny said, placing vocal emphasis on each word,

"A fucking numbers racket?"

"Apparently you didn't," I said, watching my roommate's reaction to the news.

"I feel so much like a fool," Danny got another beer and tossed me a coke,

"I should have taken the money."

"If you could turn back the clock … would you really take the money?"

"You goddamn right I would .. knowing what I know now .. in a heartbeat!"

"But that's against the law, Danny," I said, facetiously.

"I'm locked up and have nothing to show for it."

"Locked-up, Danny?" I said, pointing to our room.

Danny thought for a moment, and we both laughed loudly together.

Inmates participating in the Sober Living Program are required to use public transportation, no driving of privately owned vehicles, and no riding in privately owned vehicles.

And then there's the Garfunkel House inmate … we have assigned parking spaces.

The AG's Office had leased a brown Ford Mustang for my use. It came with a government gas card.

So this is how the privileged live!

Christmas decorations were starting to crop up. With Thanksgiving just a week away, a conglomeration of harvest-time and festive commemorations engorged the air, magnetizing San Diego towards its favorite holiday season.

Bloomberg's holiday window display said it all; Santa Claus was riding the back of a turkey through a harvesting theme into a Christmas panorama.

"Katie, get Bob Mason on a secure line," Mike called across the open office, "Herm, good... I need you to take a look at these...."

I followed Mike, almost running, to the other side of the office.

"You recognize anyone in these?" Mike had a bunch of pictures spread out on the desk he had assigned to me.

"Where'd you get these?" I asked, inspecting each picture, one by one.

"You see anybody you know?" Mike repeated, impatiently.

"Yeah ... everybody, well ... just about everybody, all cops, I don't know about this guy," I said moving a picture to the center of the desk, "Most of these guys are cops and deputies. This guy is CHP." I handed Mike a picture of Steve Shaw, a sergeant with the North County Station.

"These pictures were found by one of our agents," Mike said, walking to the coffee table.

"We don't know where the pictures were taken...."

"These two...." I said, running back to the desk, "these were taken in the lobby of the Douglas Hotel."

"Does the hotel have a basement?"

"Yeah, I've been down there."

"Is there any place in this city you don't know about?"

"Not in the downtown area, there isn't."

"Teddy…Jack, I need you on this," Mike called to two suits, "get a search warrant for this place," Mike handed one of the suits a folder.

"Listen up everybody, Herm has ID'd the location in the pictures. Frank …put together a search team and roll on this now."

The office came alive to Mike's orders, not like a cluster-fuck, but more like the Marines, a well-trained military machine.

"Herm, you gotta see this," Danny called me from the bathroom, "did you know about this raid?"

"Yeah …" I stopped to listen.

"California Landmark 121, the infamous St. Douglas Hotel is back in the news again," Edwin Whipple, late TV news, was reporting.

"Turn it up a little," I asked Danny and parked myself on the sofa next to him.

"If you remember, two years ago, the Douglas Hotel made headlines when the city's all-time largest prostitution ring was discovered there by police, operating on the grounds of this luminous state landmark.

Today, many of the officers on the 1973 raid were named in an indictment after a raid by state and federal officers. It appears that the officers were operating the state's largest book-making organization. City, county, and state employees, namely - law enforcement officers, are cooperating with authorities."

Thanksgiving dinner at Garfunkel House was much like Thanksgiving dinner at a Southern Baptist Church.

Families of the inmates were invited for the day. Wives, girlfriends, and kids had an 18-hour free run of Dwight's museum.

Herman P. Wiggins, Jr.

All the priceless antiques were put away, and the Green Corridor was roped off.

Everyone was having fun … eating .. drinking .. laughing .. and trimming the full-size tree in the great-room.

But there was no celebrating at the Shaffer home. Chief Shaffer was relieved of command from the SDPD yesterday.

Sheriff Calvin Quintanas had his job only until tomorrow …the county decided to give the Sheriff a nice Thanksgiving by postponing his dismissal until the following day.

I'm sure that gesture brought jubilee to the Quintanas' household and holiday spirit.

Chapter – 21

"ONE BLOODY MESS"

"I don't want to hear another excuse," former Mayor Dwayne David Doones said to his team of attorneys, "If you'd eliminated that problem when I told you to, none of this would've happened."

"I just knew he wouldn't survive the camp," said Attorney #2.

"He survived Vietnam … you dip-shit!" Doones said with a certain amount of aggravation and a volume close to screaming … and pointing his finger at the attorneys. "You fucked up and my dick is in the vice again."

"He'll never get to court," said Attorney #2.

"Back off," Doones said, in deep thought, "forget about Wiggins, the damage is done, what about this cop...what's his name?"

"Pineira," said Attorney #2, reading from a paper he took from his briefcase. "George T. Pineira, 18-year veteran, has a wife and seven kids."

"Goddamn corrupt cops," Doones said.

"Poor guy, probably needed the money .. you know - with seven kids and all," Attorney #1 said.

"Fuck him!" Doones shouted, "He's our problem now … he's squealing like a little trapped pig."

"The guy is just trying to make the best deal for himself, everybody is," said Attorney #1.

"Why don't you go work for them," Doones jumped to his feet .. well, as much jumping his overweight body could sustain, "Get outta here, you're fired."

"You can't fire him Sir," advised Attorney #2, "we don't work for you. Franklin, Pincer and Yepes are handling your defense and appeal…. *pro bono*, so to speak, his father is Pincer. You're broke Mr. Mayor."

"Get that smirk off your face…punk," Doones said to Attorney #1.

"Fuck you…you fat piece of shit," Attorney #1 was now on his feet, shouting and pointing his finger in Doones' face, "you pompous ass…calling that cop corrupt. He's just a guy trying to supplement a shitty salary while truly corrupt politicians like you get fatter bank accounts."

The young attorney stopped long enough to light a cigarette.

"You can't smoke in here," Doones said.

"Shut up and sit down," Attorney #1 said, continuing, "I'm good at what I do, damn good. I'm that thin pink line between…" Attorney #1 was now only inches from Doones' saggy face, speaking very slow and very low, "…. between your corrupt ass and twenty years in prison."

Former Mayor Dwayne David Doones got the point and sat quietly through the remaining minutes of the strategy meeting.

The morning traffic in San Diego is nothing like L A. or Frisco. With a population of 1,357,854 and an annual growth rate of 2.45%, a 20-minute drive from San Diego State College to downtown had augmented to 45-minutes.

But the laid-back style of San Diego and the people who came here to live that laid-back style, easily absorbed the stress of traffic ... or ... anything else that tried to park its allures on its borders. This is...CAMELOT...you know.

And that's what - being a **San Diegan** is all about. We're all here for one thing...the lifestyle.

I spent the day bouncing from one investigator's desk to another. They came from the bay area or out of state ... they had tight jaws and up-tight attitudes.

Having worked the streets, I was able to bring direction to their investigation...

They were about to meet pimps, pushers, whores and prostitutes... bag people, shop-keepers, and just down to earth street people ... people these guys never meet.

Among the people I missed, and was proud to know, was Benny —- the heroin dealer, Jennifer - the poolroom hustler, and Melissa - the prostitute.

Melissa was my training officer on the streets. We had a short thing going for a minute, or maybe it was five minutes... We would talk all night.

"You have any idea how much money these conversations cost me," Melissa would say, and then do something silly, like...fart.

"I'm a prostitute .. I'm paid well for my services," was my first lesson, "a whore wears a wedding ring."

Part of the condition of my incarceration was that I would stay away from all known criminal elements. But I was so tempted to take a walk down 5th Street.

I missed them ... they were my friends ... my family. As I think about it, they were my only friends.

The cold night air was biting at my frozen – hungry – ass. Dinner hours had passed at Garfunkel House; Denny's would have to suffice.

I was thinking about George Pineira and his dilemma. George was one of the cops who stuck by me when my head was on the chopping block. Now he and Sandy were tasting the anticipations of a long-term separation. *If I had his number, I would call*, I thought, as I entered the 94 freeway East and read the upcoming street signs.

Euclid Avenue, 925 South Euclid Avenue, I remembered his address, I should, I ate there enough times.

Sandy and George met at San Diego State College. The first time I saw Sandy was in a Logistic Management class at State. She was Miss Homecoming or something like that in her senior year. Tall, long, very long legs, and a body to match her pretty face.

George was an All-State football player, one of those big defensive linebackers with that All-American look. The chemistry between them was so strong that it was just undeniable that something was going to come of their relationship. Everyone knew they would marry and make pretty babies. Seven years… and seven pretty babies later…

I took the Euclid exit. I wanted George to know I was there for him as much as I could be, given my own predicament.

Sandy picked this four-bedroom stucco in what was once an up and coming neighborhood. As the economy started to open-up, so did the doors of white-flight.

Lower income families moved in and dropped the value of property. George and Sandy, like so many young white couples in the area, couldn't afford to move, and they were left behind.

Just as I entered the driveway, the front door flew open, two men dressed in black staggered down the stairs. One man was carrying the other who was limping and favoring his left leg. They both stopped and pointed M-16 automatic rifles in my direction.

I flung myself to the floor of the car and was showered with broken windshield glass as 15 – maybe, 20 - rounds were popped off and flying around the interior of my rented car.

I wasn't about to lie there and wait for them to come to me. I opened the front passenger door and fell face first to the ground .. that is to say .. face first into a huge pile of dog do-do.

I crawled to the front of the car, picking dog shit out of my nose and teeth and right ear. When I heard a car door close … followed by the sound and smell of burnt tire rubber … I breathed for the first time.

I instinctively reached for my .357, and remembered who I now was. The house was dark, I waited and listened for something…. anything, but there was nothing, no light…no sound.

I low crawled around the north side of the house and to the open back door.

I slithered through the door… across the service room floor … and to the door leading to the kitchen.

The place was a mess. If I remember correctly, Sandy's housekeeping skills would never have gotten the Betty Crocker Good Housekeeping Award, but this was more than Sandy could or would have tolerated.

I realized this was the result of a hasty search.

A car passing on the street illuminated the living room. I could see a pair of feet just inches from the door. They were lying sideways and not moving.

I crawled to the door and saw two bodies, one near the kitchen wall and the other sitting next to the front door.

I didn't recognize the guy by the door, but the one closest to me was George Pineira. I shook his feet to see what response I could get, there was none.

From the lights of passing cars, I could see an M-16 lying across the lap of the man sitting next to the front door.

I pried the .45 from George's right hand and crawled across the floor to the man with the M-16. I pulled the M-16 away and checked his pulse. There was none.

I patted his limp body to check for other weapons, there were none.

I crawled back to George's body and saw another body lying in the hallway.

This guy was laying face down with an M-16 lying at his feet. I searched him and retrieved a .38 from an ankle holster.

Blood was everywhere, I was soaked from head to feet, and still had dog shit up my nose and in my ear.

"George.... can you hear me George?" I whispered in his ear and checked his pulse again, there was a pulse, very faint and intermittent.

Blood was gushing from his left upper leg. I applied direct pressure using a tablecloth that was lying on the floor next to George. Using the cord from a broken lamp, I placed a tourniquet approximately four inches above the two bullet wounds.

George coughed, "George...George can you hear me?" I called.

He tightened his grip on my arm.

"George, it's me, Herman."

"Herm?" He opened his eyes for the first time, "Herm... what the fuck are you doing here?"

"Just stopped by to say hi."

"Well…?."

"Well what?" I could see George wanting to close his eyes.

"Well…. say hi." George had trouble forcing out the words.

"Hi George, how the fuck have you been?"

"Not too fucking good, Herm, I think I've been shot."

"A couple of times." I said, checking his pulse again, "I stopped the bleeding, but you've lost a lot of blood."

George was fading in and out, his eyes were rolling back in his head.

"George…wake up," I shook his shoulders, "you can't go to sleep, I'll call for help, where's the phone? George….wake-up, stay with me here, listen, you have got to fight this, you can make it, help me George, fight the urge to sleep."

His eyes opened, "…you still here Good-Buddy….?"

"Where's the phone?" I shouted.

"On the wall, in the kitchen, next to this stove," George pointed.

I found the phone, it was dead. I checked the master bedroom and found another phone on the dresser, it was also dead.

"George, you still with me?"

"I'm here, where the fuck do you think I'm going?" his voice was weakening.

"Where's Sandy and the kids?"

"In San Francisco with my brother," he coughed, "I figured something like this would happen."

"Good thinking."

"They were cops .. cops came after me," George was squeezing my hand harder, "I knew those guys, we drank and partied together."

"Cops? SDPD cops?" I asked. His pulse was the same.

"Dave McMillan, Larry Rivers, Andy Sherman..." George said. I loosened the tourniquet. "....and Brad Warr."

His voice was fading, in direct proportion to his fading pulse.

"I think I hit one," his words were now coming with increased strain.

"You got two ... Hot-shot."

"I know .. that's Andy at the door."

I checked the man at the door for ID and found a badge and police ID in the name of Andy C. Sherman.

"The guy in the hallway also has a police ID and badge," I called to George, "this guy is Dave (nmn) McMillan."

"Dave is Sandy's first cousin."

"What the fuck have you gotten yourself into George?" I asked, tightening the tourniquet.

"Big money was on the line .. I fucked up. The money, it was just coming in. My son...Rickey...he was born with a hole in his heart, the hospital bills, they were killing us. We were in hock up to our nose. Then this came along, we paid off our bills, we were moving next weekend ... Sandy found a much larger house in El Cajon, near where you used to live. The money was there, my kid needed it.

I tried to quit … but the money kept coming."

"Hey…stay with me George, I've got to get help for you. What's your neighbors names?"

"My neighbors? Don't get my neighbors involved in this."

"You need help, I have to get to a phone."

"The <u>Howes</u> on the left and the <u>Sloanes</u> on the right."

Chapter – 22

HONOR THY FATHER'S WORDS

"Mr. Todd, have you heard from Mr. Wiggins tonight?" Dwight Ackley asked when Danny answered the faint knock at our room door.

"No I haven't," Danny said with an apologetic shrug, "it's not like Herm to be late.

I will have to report this violation. I don't want to get Mr. Wiggins in any trouble, so I'll hold off as long as I can. If you know or hear anything, please keep me informed."

* * * * * * * * * * * *

I started out the door…. stopped, and thought of every horror movie I'd ever seen where the bad guys comes alive, and the weapon's laying there waiting for them to use again.

I put the .38 in my belt, strapped the M-16s on each shoulder, and carried the .45 in my hand.

"Left HOWE…right SLOANE… or was it right – HOWE and left – SLOANE?"

I ran south across the lawn toward the light brown house.

"Mrs. Sloane," I said to the elderly woman answering the door.

"No!" She snapped.

"Mrs. Howe?" I tried again.

"Yes," she said smiling, her voice much softer now.

"I need to use your phone," I shouted.

The lady turned the light on to see who she was talking to, and as soon as the light illuminated the front porch she started screaming. She screamed so loud it could have brought the two stiffs next-door back to life.

Mrs. Howe slammed the door … I grabbed the doorknob … turned it, and threw my shoulder and weight into the door. The lady didn't have time to flip the lock.

The door flew open knocking Mrs. Howe to the floor.

"Everybody stay cool," I said to the four people sitting at the long dinner table,

"I know how this must look to you, a Black man kicking your door in, carrying two M-16s on his shoulder, brandishing a .45, and covered with blood. To say nothing of this dog shit up my nose – and – in my ear," I picked at my nose again. "The police officer who lives next door… has been shot … he's loosing a lot of blood. I need to use your phone?"

"Over here," said the lady sitting at the far end of the table.

I picked up the phone and dialed 9-1-1.

"Drop the guns," I heard, and looked up to see a skinny senior citizen male pointing a double-barrel shotgun at my head.

"Sir…. I am not here to harm any of you…."

"Drop the guns," he repeated, sighting down the long barrels.

"OK…. I'm putting the guns down," I leaned over to put my arsenal in the nearby chair.

The nervous senior citizen fired the shotgun, blowing away the door behind me.

I dropped to the floor and waited for the old fellow to regain control of his emotions.

"Operator.... hello.... this is police officer Wiggins," I continued talking, "Detective Pineira has been shot. He's at 925 South Euclid Avenue, we need help, NOW!"

"What is the phone number you're calling from...Sir?"

"What's this number?" I shouted, holding up the phone.

"263-6114," the first-lady of the house shouted back.

"I heard her Sir, 263-6114," the 911 operator repeated, "we have units rolling now."

"I am so sorry to have disturbed your dinner party," I said, handing the lady of the house the phone, "please direct the police next door if they should call back."

I got to my feet and checked on the old fellow with the shotgun ... who had been knocked to the floor by the big gun's recall.

"You OK Sir?" I helped him to his feet, "Again...I apologize to all of you, thanks for the use of your phone."

I ran from the house carrying only the .45.

"Police," a voice shouted, and the spotlights of four patrol cars had me surrounded, *"drop the weapon."*

I threw the .45 to my right .. in plain sight of the army of officers drawing down on me.

"Get down on the ground," another voice of authority ordered.

And I complied.

Flashlights and light-brown uniforms approached my now motionless body.

"Wiggins, what the fuck are you doing here?" I heard a familiar voice ask.

"I stopped by to check on George," I said, looking up into the face of my first field-training officer, David Lancaster.

"Get up," David ordered, lightly nudging my leg with his foot.

"We've got two dead and one in bad shape," an officer called from the front door, "looks like they're all cops."

"Herman.... what can you tell me about all of this?" Lancaster asked.

There was something about his voice and the look on his face that alarmed me.

Four cops were sent to kill a brother cop: Two dead .. two got away .. and their mark is hanging on by the threads of one breath at a time.

And here I am: A known rogue-cop ... a convicted cop ... in a place I should not be ... covered with blood and dog shit ... looking up the barrels of guns held by police officers.

"Junior... you can always trust a police officer, whenever you get in a mess, call the police, that's what they're there for... to help you." My father's words were ringing through my head.

But this was not one of those times to honor thy father's words, I felt trusting the cops in this case could be very hazardous to my health.

"Did Pineira say anything to you," Lancaster asked.

"No," I lied, "he never regained consciousness."

"Are you sure?"

"Yes... I'm sure," I said, and I felt he knew I was lying.

Herman P. Wiggins, Jr.

"Detective .. may I speak to you over here?" A baby-faced patrol officer said to Lancaster.

"Sure," Dave answered, as the two officers moved to the rear of the patrol car I was sitting in.

"I just walked in on something that looked strange to me," the young officer whispered, "That officer over there," he pointed, "the one in black ...I think he was trying to smother detective Pineira."

"Are you sure?" the sound in David's voice was sincere.

"Yeah...I'm sure that's what he was doing."

"Ok, I'll take care of this."

David started walking towards the officer in black, the one the young officer had pointed out.

"Detective Lancaster," I called at a whisper, "who's that officer?"

"Larry," Dave said.

"Larry Rivers?" I asked.

"Yeah, you know him?"

"David, I need to talk to you," I motioned for him to join me in the patrol car, "keep an eye on him."

"What's going on Herm?"

"I lied when you asked if Pineira had said anything to me."

"Why?"

I took a deep breath and thought of all George Pineira had told me.

"I don't know whom to trust … Pineira did talk to me … he gave me the names of the four cops who shot up his place. He took out the two in the house and two got away. When I drove up, I saw two men running from the house, one was wounded and being carried by the other, they were wearing black, like what Rivers is wearing."

"Did you get a look at their faces?"

"No, I was ducking a volley of 7.62-mm rounds. That's my car over there, the dead one … the one with the windows shot out."

I spoke slowly, watching for any revealing changes of expression in Lancaster's verbalizations. I could be wrong, but I felt I could trust him.

"Larry," Dave called to the officer in black, "I need to talk to you."

"About what?" Larry moved towards the street.

"I just need to talk to you for a moment."

Before Detective David Lancaster could react, Larry Rivers drew his revolver and pumped two rounds into David's chest. He was dead before he hit the ground.

As Officer Rivers ran from the yard, two uniformed officers opened fire, dropping the corrupt cop before he reached the street.

Chapter – 23

A LONG OVERDUE LAUGH

"Heard you had an exciting night," Mike Mattox greeted me the next morning.

"Exciting night and morning," I answered, heading for the coffee pot, "I haven't slept in over 24 hours."

"Look at you," Mike said, and the office stopped doing what they were doing and looked in my direction, "all covered with blood … you look like shit … what's that brown stuff up your nose?"

"Shit…. dog shit," I tried picking my nose again.

"Go get cleaned-up, you're stinking up the office."

"I need a car, mine got killed."

"Is this the way you were as a cop?"

"Pretty much so, seems like this kind of *shit* just follows me."

"I would have hated being one of your watch commanders. I can only imagine the paperwork you generated for them," Mike said, tossing me his keys.

"True…. but they never complained about having a boring day," I took the cup of coffee and keys and left for the day. First stop…THE SHOWER.

Hearings … Meetings … Depositions … Testimonies… and Luncheons — Meeting one attorney in the morning, and two in the afternoon.

Most nights I didn't get back to Garfunkel House until 8:30 or 9:00. I rarely ate dinner there anymore ... and was on the road many mornings before their breakfast hour.

The grueling drill continued until the week before Christmas.

The Governor's appointed task force had probed into the depth of every crack and crevice of municipal and county government.

Musical chairs was the game of choice ...new faces were replacing old ones.

One old face decided to pack up and leave. Only problem is, he decided to take the window.

A clean sweep of city hall brought a bright new hope to San Diego's future.

Millions of embezzled city and county bucks were returned to treasury books, some mysteriously.

On the 28th of December, at 1645-hours, a four-man, eight-woman Grand Jury posted their findings. Twenty-eight indictments were handed down...

including: six for former Mayor Dwayne David Doones and the Doonesbury Machine ... for: mail fraud — racketeering — money laundering — and conspiracy_to bribe a Federal Magistrate.

Detective David Lancaster didn't make it out of George Pineira's front yard.

DOA at the scene: Bull's eye...two shots...center heart.

Officer Brad Warr was arrested at Holy Mountain Hospital .. he turned states evidence and is doing 15 to 20 at Ironwood State Prison for attempted 187 – Murder.

Yeah.... George made it, he got fucked up pretty bad, but with a little TLC from Sandy, he's going to be OK. Lucky son-of-a-bitch ... got away with a slap on the wrist and a forced career change, no jail time.

"Mr. Wiggins," Dwight handed me a stack of phone messages, "one in particular there... a Mr. Mitchell, he's called about 12 times."

"My attorney, Lewis Mitchell," I took the messages and went to my empty room.

Danny Todd was released last week. We had our **hoop-la** party at the Do-Drop-Inn in El Cajon ... Why he was so attracted to that dive, I'll never understand.

"The Do-Drop-Inn is the type of place people like me would never see, except in movies," Danny explained on our last night together, "I just saw this movie, **Looking For Mr. Goodbar,** with Diane Keaton and Tuesday Weld.

This is the type of bar where Diane Keaton would pick up her victims. Hey...maybe we'll get lucky enough to be the victims of a couple of Diane Keaton and Tuesday Weld look-alikes."

"I'm going to miss you...you sick puppy," I said, right - arm around my jail-house buddy's shoulders ... sitting at a bar... sucking on a couple of *cold-ones.*

"Let's keep in touch," Danny said, between gulps.

"Can't promise you that ... Good-Buddy. Don't know what road I'll be traveling from here."

My after-jail life was something I knew I had to look at .. just didn't have the time.

Now that I think about it, where do I go from here? I'll cross that road when I get to it.

Uncle Tom's Hanging Tree

"Lewis... Herman here, heard you been calling," I said from the phone in my room, "What's up?"

"You are," Lewis' voice was bubbly, "up and out."

"I know there's a hidden message in this riddle, but I think it's over my head."

"Pack up...the judge is releasing you tomorrow. I need you in Department 21 at 9:30, meet me in the hall."

Packing, for a person like me, was no extensive task. A brown J.C. Penny's shopping bag was more than enough luggage to carry my worldly possessions.

"Herman....you're looking good."

"Thank you, Your Honor...you're about as ugly as ever."

Judge Green and I enjoyed a couple of cups of coffee and a long overdue laugh together.

"Where's my attorney?"

"Lewis was here earlier, he and Thompson from the Probation Department worked through all the paperwork, dotting *i*'s and crossing *t*'s."

Judge Green handed me a stack of papers.

"Just sign here and you're a free man."

I looked over the legal documents as if I knew what I was reading.

"I'm the one who sentenced you," the Judge handed me a pen, "I asked Lewis and Thompson to leave us to meet alone here in chambers."

"Ed ... I have no grudge with you," I signed the two papers and handed the judge his pen.

"Keep it."

"Something to remember this moment by?" I smiled.

"Something like that," Ed smiled, "I hated what I had to do to you."

"You did your job Ed …I would not have expected anything less."

The papers were a court order from the Superior Court of the State of California. Case# CR-23248.

Order: ***Dismissing accusations against probationer (sec: 1204-pc).***

"I entered a plea of not guilty on your behalf, it's all over, where are you going from here?" Ed asked.

"I don't know, this got sprung on me quite suddenly. I know I should have been thinking about it … don't have a home or any family, so-to-speak-of. No one to return to. Everything I own is in this brown bag, no car…well, I still have the rental from the AG's Office. Think I'll hang on to it for a while. I'll call them in a couple of months and tell them where to pick it up."

"Will you ever change, Herm?"

"Hope not…. I'm having too much fun."

"How do you live like that … from one adventure to another?"

"It's all I know, Judge."

"Haven't you ever wanted to settle down and start a family?"

"Tried it once…bored me shitless … anyway .. I've got time for that if I ever want to try the family thing again."

We both got to our feet at the same time … we shook hands and embraced.

"Promise me you'll keep in touch."

"Can't promise that Judge, when I move on … I move on… you know what I mean."

"No, I don't…but …good luck anyway. Herman…watch your back out there."

Shit…. I hate it when people tell me that.

This was the day I had been waiting to arrive for over a year. Like Vietnam, working the justice system was an experience. Neither would I care to repeat, but each has made me stronger for what's up the road.

The warm January sun felt good on my face … there wasn't a cloud in the sky, there wasn't a care in my heart.

"Are you finished with that," I was talking with the wino parked in front of the courthouse.

"You want a drink young man?" queried the wino with the empty bottle.

"No, I just want to spin it."

"Like in *spin-the-bottle*?" The wino puckered up.

"Yeah…" I said placing the wine bottle on the ground and giving it a quick clockwise spin.

"It's facing me … that means I get a kiss?"

"Sorry old fellow, you're not my type, the bottle is pointing north."

North it will be……Los Angeles or San Francisco or maybe….Canada.

"Mr. Wiggins," a woman called from a side door at the courthouse, "are you Herman Wiggins?"

"Yes," I answered reluctantly.

"There's a phone call for you in here."

"Officer Herman Phillip Wiggins, Jr." the soft male voice on the other end of the line said, *"surely you remember me."*

"Who is this?"

"Let's say it's...The Doctor."

"Doctor...who?"

"You said you would never forget me, OFFICER. W-I-G-G-I-N-S ... I'll never forget you."

"Who the fuck is this?" I shouted, gaining the attention of everyone in the small office.

"This is your friend," the voice continued to tug-at-me.

And there was a long silence, the longest and loudest silence I have ever experienced.

"This is Dr. Tomiko Sciortino."

I drove north as fast as I could ... not running away, but just putting as much of my past behind me ... as quickly as I could.

Through the rearview mirror I watched the San Diego skyline fading, and I thought... *"Will this extraordinary odyssey ever end for me?"*

THE END